# Writing Skills in Practice

*of related interest*

**Communication Skills in Practice**
A Practical Guide for Health Professionals
*Diana Williams*
1 85302 232 2

**Advocacy Skills for Health and Social Care Professionals**
*Neil Bateman*
1 85302 865 7

**Boring Records?**
Communication, Speech and Writing in Social Work
*Katie Prince*
1 85302 325 6

**Negotiation for Health and Social Service Professionals**
*Keith Fletcher*
1 85302 549 6

**Staff Supervision in a Turbulent Environment**
Managing Process and Task in Front-line Services
*Lynette Hughes and Paul Pengelly*
1 85302 327 2

# Writing Skills in Practice
## A Practical Guide for Health Professionals

*Diana Williams*

Jessica Kingsley Publishers
London and Philadelphia

First published in the United Kingdom in 2002
by Jessica Kingsley Publishers Ltd
116 Pentonville Road
London N1 9JB, England
and
325 Chestnut Street
Philadelphia, PA 19106, USA
*www.jkp.com*

Copyright © 2002 Diana Williams

**Library of Congress Cataloging in Publication Data**
Williams, Diana, 1957-
    Writing skills in practice : a practical guide for health professionals / Diana Williams.
    p.cm.
    Includes bibliographical references and index.
    ISBN 1-85302-649-2 (alk paper)
    1. Medical writing. 2. Communication in medicine. I. Title.

R119.W49 2002
808'.06661--dc21                                                        2002021524

**British Library Cataloguing in Publication Data**
A CIP catalogue record for this book is available from the British Library

ISBN 1 85302 649 2

Printed and Bound in Great Britain by
Athenaeum Press, Gateshead, Tyne and Wear

# Contents

Introduction 9

The Nature of Written Communication 11

Communicating Effectively through the Written Word 13

**Part One: Writing for Clinical Practice 17**

*1 Purpose of Written Material 21*
*2 How to Record Information 29*
*3 The Legal Framework 34*

Clinical Skills in Context:
*4 Record Keeping 43*
*5 Letters and Reports 71*
*6 Information Leaflets For Clients 93*

**Part Two: Writing for Teaching and Learning 119**

*7 Writing as an Aid to Learning 123*
*8 Preparing Materials for Teaching 140*

Teaching and Learning Skills in Context:
*9 Note-taking 153*
*10 Essays 167*
*11 Assessment 187*
*12 Dissertations 194*
*13 Research Projects 204*

# Part Three: Writing for Publication 223

*14 Developing an Idea 227*
*15 Managing Your Time Effectively 233*
*16 Determining Your Style 247*
*17 Getting the Best Out of Your Personal Computer 254*
*18 Presenting Your Work 259*
*19 Protecting Your Rights 270*

## Publication Skills in Context:

*20 Journal Articles 275*
*21 Books 288*
*22 Articles for the Media 302*

## References 316

## Index 320

References 316

Index 320

# List of Figures

| | | |
|---|---|---|
| Figure 4.1 | Summary of record keeping at key stages in the care process | 69–70 |
| Figure 5.1 | Standard format of a letter | 75–76 |
| Figure 9.1 | Sequential notes | 156 |
| Figure 9.2 | Spider web notes | 158 |
| Figure 9.3 | Pattern notes | 160 |
| Figure 11.1 | A mind map | 189 |
| Figure 13.1 | A vertical bar chart | 212 |
| Figure 13.2 | A horizontal bar chart | 212 |
| Figure 13.3 | A multiple bar chart | 213 |
| Figure 13.4 | A proportional bar chart | 214 |
| Figure 13.5 | A pie chart | 214 |
| Figure 13.6 | A histogram | 215–216 |
| Figure 13.7 | A frequency polygon | 216 |
| Figure 13.8 | A line graph | 217 |
| Figure 13.9 | A scattergram | 218 |
| Figure 15.1 | A planning sheet | 236 |
| Figure 15.2 | A daily timetable | 239 |
| Figure 15.3 | A daily activity record | 242 |
| Figure 15.4 | Extract from a completed daily activity record | 243 |
| Figure 22.1 | A query letter | 308 |
| Figure 22.2 | A guide to analysing the content, approach and style of media articles | 313–314 |

Dedicated with love
to Elizabeth May Williams

# Introduction

One of the main methods of communication within the health service is the written word, whether this is in the form of clinical notes, reports or letters. An increasing emphasis is being placed on improving and maintaining the quality of such communications. This means the written output of clinicians is under more rigorous scrutiny than ever before.

The first part of this book offers practical guidance in developing the effective writing skills required in everyday clinical practice. It will be useful for students learning about clinical documentation and for practitioners wishing to review their writing practices.

Training, teaching and continuing education are essential in the development of a skilled workforce in the health service. All clinicians are involved in this process, first as students then later as experienced clinicians mentoring or training others. The second part of this book addresses the various writing demands arising in such teaching and learning contexts. It covers topics as far-ranging as effective note-taking, preparing teaching materials and writing up research.

The final part of the book is dedicated to writing for publication. There are many opportunities for health professionals to place their written work in the public arena. Writing books and journal articles provides an opportunity for disseminating information, sharing best practice and stimulating debate. It contributes to the knowledge base of the profession and helps maintain the dynamic nature of the care process. Becoming a published author is also a great personal achievement, and this section offers advice on how, what and where to publish.

This book is intended for use by a variety of health care workers that includes therapists, health visitors, nurses and general practitioners.

**How to use this book**

The book is designed to give the reader easy access to information. A breakdown of topic areas is provided at the beginning of each part, so that the reader can quickly identify sections of interest.

Alternatively, the reader can refer to the summary points at the end of each chapter. These provide a brief guide to the content of each subsection.

# The Nature of Written Communication

The written word, like spoken communication, is used for a variety of functions. Just a few of these are listed below:

- to instruct
- to inform
- to express ideas or an opinion
- to direct
- to debate and discuss
- to persuade
- to develop logical ideas
- to describe
- to entertain
- to hypothesise
- to summarise
- to list.

All of the above can be equally applied to spoken language. So what is it about the nature of the written word that often gives it preference over speech?

- ◊ The written word offers a more enduring form of communication than the spoken word. This makes it an ideal choice for recording information, so that it can be referred to repeatedly and preserved over a long period of time.

- ◊ Duplicates of letters, reports and other documents are easily produced. This allows sharing of information amongst a range of people who do not have to be present to witness the original communication.

◊ The writer has more time to organise his or her thoughts and assemble complex facts and figures. There is time to review the intended message and redraft if necessary.

◊ Writing is often the first choice when formality is required. A formal letter or report will indicate to the recipient the seriousness of the matter under discussion.

It is important to remember that writing differs significantly from spoken language. In speech, additional meaning and information are often conveyed through the body language or vocal characteristics of the speaker. This element of communication is absent from the written message. The writer needs to use skill and creativity in order to achieve the same depth of meaning and nuance as the spoken message.

Also, text is often read separately in time and place from the people and events to which it relates. There is a lack of immediate feedback about the level of the reader's interest, understanding and involvement. The written word must make sense away from the context to which it refers. The onus is on the writer to provide all the necessary information required by the reader, and to modify vocabulary and language to meet the anticipated needs of the reader.

Despite some drawbacks, the written word continues to be one of the main methods of communication within the health service. The next chapter identifies the key elements in communicating effectively using writing.

# Communicating Effectively through the Written Word

In its most simple definition, an 'effective written communication' is one that achieves its purpose. In order to make this happen the writer needs to think about:

- o the objective or aim of writing
- o the intended audience
- o the message
- o how the message is phrased
- o how the message is presented
- o access to the message.

*The objective:* Writers must be clear about what they want their writing to achieve. The content, format and presentation will all depend on the purpose of the message.

*The audience:* The needs, interests and knowledge of the reader must be anticipated and the writing planned accordingly.

*The message:* This is about the content or meaning that the writer wants to convey to the reader.

*How the message is phrased:* The choice of vocabulary and the way in which the message is phrased will vary according to the purpose, the context and the reader.

*How the message is presented:* The layout and the format of the text plays an important part in attracting the reader. It also helps to organise the information and thereby increases the readability of the piece.

*Access to the message:* The writer must consider how and when the reader will have access to the written message. So circulation lists must be considered when writing reports, whereas methods of distribution are important when writing information leaflets for clients.

## Characteristics of effective written communication

There is nothing magical about the following criteria for effective writing skills; all would be easily elicited from any group of professionals. However, it is still worthwhile to reiterate them as a reminder of the basics of good writing. In addition to this despite being well known they are not always applied in everyday situations. This has sometimes resulted in poor standards of written communication leading to inadequate record keeping, complaints by clients and clinical errors. It is hoped that this list will serve as a useful reminder and prompt some reflection on the writing process and its outcome.

An effective written communication is:

   ○ Engaging

It is essential that the writing gets noticed in the first place. In some cases, the way that the message is delivered ensures this, for example a letter is posted to a specific person. However, in health promotion, engaging the attention of the reader becomes paramount. The next step is to ensure that the message is of enough interest to prompt the reader to continue.

   ○ Comprehensive

The message is complete, and the reader is not left feeling there is something missing.

   ○ Concise

The reader will want to access the key points with the minimum amount of effort. Writing therefore needs to be concise and extraneous material removed.

   ○ Relevant

The information contained in the message must be consistent with both the writer's intention and the requirements of the reader.

   ○ Appropriate in tone

The tone of the writing must be compatible with its purpose and the context in which it is being used.

- ○ Consistent with other communications

The message should not contradict other communications, unless this is the specific purpose in order to rectify an error.

- ○ Legible

A clear text is a simple but fundamental requirement if the message is to be understood and misunderstandings avoided.

- ○ Timely

The message needs to be received at the right time for it to achieve its purpose and meet the needs of the reader. A delay in receiving information is often a cause of complaint. However, sometimes information may be given too early. For example, clients vary in the types of information they need at different points in the care process.

- ○ Logical

The content of the message needs to make sense to the reader. The writer needs to organise information into a logical sequence, and make explicit the links between facts.

- ○ Accurate

Incorrect information can mislead the reader and cause confusion. It will also affect the credibility of the writer and may cast doubt on the validity of judgements in other matters.

- ○ Well presented

The way information is presented to the reader has an impact on readability and comprehension. Providing structure by arranging text in paragraphs and supplying headings helps to organise information. Well laid out text is also more inviting to the reader.

- ○ Accessible

This is about making sure that the right people have access to documents at the right time. There is no point having an excellent piece of documentation if it is unavailable.

## PART ONE

# Writing for Clinical Practice

# Writing for Clinical Practice

An essential but sometimes overlooked component of clinical skills is a competence in writing. Written documentation is used extensively by clinicians to plan and deliver the most appropriate and effective care for the client. With the increase in litigation it is also important that clinicians keep a written record of the quality and extent of this care. The Department of Health, in its circular 'For the Record' (NHS Executive 1999), stresses the importance of adequate record keeping, and reminds us that information management is a professional activity. Good quality notes are seen as a reflection of a careful and thoughtful practitioner.

The main section of this part outlines the reasons for the various forms of documentation, and offers advice on improving standards of record keeping. The legal framework within which information management operates is also reviewed and its implications for clinicians discussed.

The final section offers advice on three specific types of written communication commonly used in clinical practice – record keeping, correspondence (in the form of letters and reports) and information leaflets for clients.

## Purpose of written material

Definition of a personal health record. Purpose of clinical documentation and information leaflets for clients.

## How to record information

Guidelines on recording clinical information.

## The legal framework

Accountability. Use and protection of information. Access to and retention of health records.

18

# Clinical skills in context

### Record Keeping

Setting up a personal health record. Recording assessment and intervention. Writing treatment objectives and out-comes. Dealing with discharge.

### Letters and Reports

Definitions. Preparing, planning and drafting documents. Summaries of key content for common types of letters and reports.

### Information Leaflets for Clients

Preparing your material. Delivering the message. Writing for special client groups. Producing your material. Evaluation of materials.

# 1

# Writing for Clinical Practice
## Purpose of Written Material

Writing is one of the principal modes of communication in any health organisation. It is used to convey information both within the health team, and from the team to clients, other professionals and organisations, hence the vast array of documents generated on a daily basis by health workers.

### Personal health records

The majority of written communications in any health service are related directly to the care and management of the client. This information is organised into individual records specially created for this purpose. They will usually include assessment forms, laboratory reports, referral letters, progress notes and drug sheets.

Clinical notes compiled for a specific client may be referred to as casenotes, medical notes or as a personal health record. They are either in a manual form, where information is recorded on paper, or, increasingly, in electronic form, where information is held on computer. The term personal health records will be used here to refer to such notes.

Personal health records help:

◊ To facilitate the delivery of care to the client.

The primary purpose of a health record is to assist in the planning and delivery of the most appropriate care for the client. The information contained within it helps the clinician in establishing the needs of the client and identifying appropriate intervention, whether that is medical treatment, therapy or nursing care.

◊ To ensure continuity of care.

Clinical notes provide a way for colleagues to share information. They are a record of the current situation with the client, and contain the details of his or her condition at that time. A clinician at any stage in the care process will know what information has been gathered and how that has been acted upon.

Information about previous contacts will also be contained within the notes. This means that the clinician is able to refer back to the client's clinical history. This helps in focusing subsequent investigations and examinations and ensuring continuity of care.

◊   To provide documentary evidence of contact with a specific client.

Clinical records provide written evidence that a service has actually been delivered. Health professionals are able to show that they have discharged their duty of care by keeping complete and timely records. This is particularly important in cases of litigation or occasions where payment for clinical activity is required.

◊   To provide documentary evidence of the nature, extent and quality of care.

As well as verifying that a service was delivered to a client, clinical records will also show the nature and extent of those contacts. The details of clinical care for a client can be compared with standards set locally, nationally and by the relevant professional body.

◊   To assure and improve quality of care.

One way of measuring the quality of the care and treatment provided for a client is to audit the record of that care. Auditing notes will help to indicate whether guidelines and standards relating to clinical practice are applied consistently by the health professional. Comparisons can also be made between members in a team and between different teams.

◊   To support the clinician's clinical decision making.

Clinical records at their most basic level are an aide-mémoire – a reminder to the clinician of the pertinent facts. This data is vital if the clinician is to make appropriate clinical decisions.

The notes made by the clinician will also demonstrate the rationale underpinning his or her clinical decision making. They will show the steps he or she has taken to determine the client's clinical need, and what actions were initiated to meet these needs. They will help confirm that these actions were, first of all, necessary and, second, adequate to meet the needs and the expectations of the client.

◊ To support the development of evidence-based practice through research.

Health records contain an abundance of data about the presentation and progression of various illnesses, treatment regimes and clinical outcomes. Here are just some of the uses to which researchers can put this information:

- ○ detection of risk factors
- ○ measuring clinical outcomes
- ○ determining the effect of client education on compliance
- ○ gathering statistics about the incidence and prevalence of certain diseases in different population groups.

◊ To provide an effectively managed service.

Not all of the ways in which client information is used are directly clinical in nature. The data contained in health records is also of importance in achieving effective health care administration (NHS Executive 1999) – so the recording of client contacts delivered by extra contractual services would be vital for financing purposes. Paperwork also needs to be provided to account for the use of resources. The provision of incontinence pads, for example, should correspond to the size of the caseload and the individual needs of the clients as documented by the clinician. Such information is essential if services are to be managed effectively on a day-to-day basis, and appropriate plans made for the future.

◊ To provide a systematic way of organising information.

Personal health records are a way of organising what can be a large amount of information in a form that is readily available to the clinician.

## Letters and reports

### Letters

Letters provide a formal method of liaison between professionals. They provide:

- ○ a way of communicating the client's needs – for example, referring a client for specialist or alternative treatment

- ○ a method of informing others about the management of the client and the outcomes of that management

- ○ a permanent record, therefore being of use as documentary evidence

- ○ a source of reference or aide-mémoire for the receiver

- ○ a confirmation of a previous spoken communication such as a conversation or a telephone call

- ○ a way of communicating with people who are not contactable through other means.

## Reports

Clinical reports are a way of conveying detailed information about specific clients. Reports are suitable for communicating information about a client that is too complex and lengthy for a letter. A report format may also be stipulated in certain circumstances such as expert witness reports for court.

Reports help the clinician to:

- ○ convey information about the assessment and management of a client

- ○ explain the clinical needs of a client

- ○ summarise the key information about a client's health needs

- ○ provide documentary evidence for the client's personal health record

- ○ persuade others to take action by highlighting the impact of the client's condition on his or her quality of life

- ○ influence the clinical decision making of other health professionals

- ○ inform others of recommendations about the care and management of the client.

Clinicians use the information in reports from other health professionals to:

- gain a greater understanding of the needs of the client in a specific area
- help focus their investigations or examinations
- assist in a differential diagnosis
- rule out any other health problems or disabilities
- gain an idea of the client's progress
- help make a decision, for example, about the feasibility of the client living independently.

## Written information for clients

Health service users are increasingly expressing a desire for more information about a variety of general, administrative and clinical issues (Coulter, Entwistle and Gilbert 1998). Providing information in a written form is one way of meeting this need.

The nature of the written word gives it a number of advantages over other ways of communicating with the client. Information is provided in a readily accessible form, which the clients are able to take away with them. They are then able to choose at what time and how often they refer to it. There is also the opportunity to provide more information in greater depth than would be feasible during the usual clinical interview.

Written information helps:

◊ To prevent illness and promote a healthy lifestyle.

Providing the client with leaflets about the symptoms and risk factors associated with an illness encourages self-care. The client has the facts to help him or her identify the early signs of disease. The leaflets encourage a healthy lifestyle by highlighting risk factors and offering advice on how to reduce these. Publishing information in this way can also help to legitimise the concerns and anxieties a client might have about a specific problem. The client is then more likely to seek advice.

◊ To improve the client's, family's and carer's experience of health care services.

Clients want and need information that will help them anticipate and understand the health care process.

Information that helps orientate the client is easily presented in a written form, which can be sent prior to the client's appointment. It might include details such as:

- location and transport arrangements
- clinic contact numbers
- instructions for making and attending appointments
- the names of key members of the health care team
- the presence of students and the client's rights in relation to this
- a description of the way in which the clinic or ward is administered.

Clients benefit from being prepared physically, mentally and emotionally for investigations and intervention. Information about what to expect and how to prepare and a description of how they might feel at different stages in the care process are all-important. For example, a booklet prepared for women about to undergo hysterectomy was found to reduce post-operative pain and distress (Young and Humphrey 1985).

◊ To involve clients in the decision making process.

Many clients want to be actively involved in making decisions about their care. Written information is one way of helping to explain to them the risks and benefits of various treatment options. Clients are then able to make informed choices not only about how to treat but also whether to treat at all. Clients who share in the decision making process in this way are more likely to be satisfied with the clinician–client relationship and comply with treatment regimes.

◊ To increase the effectiveness of clinical care.

Written information helps the client to understand (Ley 1988) and retain more of the spoken message (Ellis *et al.* 1979). The use of written materials is therefore likely to improve the effectiveness of communication within the clinical interview. In addition, clients are able to use the same information when explaining issues to family and carers.

◊ To ensure equality of access.

If clients are to be proactive in meeting their health needs, they need to know about the services that are available at a local, regional and national level. This is particularly important for client groups who may have English as a second language or for those groups who hold a special status such as refugees. Leaflets and posters can also be used to increase awareness of services that are directed at specific client groups, for example a family planning service for teenagers.

◊ To involve the client, family and carers in policy making.

More initiatives are being taken to involve users in policy making for health services in the future. In order for these users to be effective in making contributions, they need to know something about the health needs of the whole community and not just their own requirements. Again written materials are a useful way of disseminating such information.

---

## Summary Points

- Writing is one of the principal modes of communication in any health organisation.

- The majority of written communications in any health service are related directly to the care and management of the client.

- Personal health records help:

  - to facilitate the delivery of care to the client

  - to ensure continuity of care

  - to achieve effective health care administration

  - to assure and improve quality of care.

- Personal health records are important documentary proof that a service was delivered and of the nature, extent and quality of that care.

- Letters and reports provide a formal method of liaison between professionals and others, such as the client, family, carers and other agencies.

- ○ Clients want more information, and providing written materials is one way of meeting this need.

- ○ Written information can help:

  - ○ to prevent illness and promote a healthy lifestyle

  - ○ to improve the client's, family's and carer's experience of health care services

  - ○ to involve clients in the decision making process, and increase the effectiveness of clinical care.

# 2

# How to Record Information

The information contained in health records is essential to the planning and delivery of care to the client. It is also important data for health service management and administration. Information needs to be accurate, complete, relevant and accessible if it is to be of use to the health professional. It is therefore essential that the quality of record keeping be maintained to the highest standard.

Information must be:

- accurate
- relevant
- complete
- accessible.

The way in which information is recorded must be:

- objective
- specific
- logical
- clear
- timely.

◊ Accurate

Accuracy is a fundamental requirement when recording information in a personal health record. Personal data should be accurate and up to date (Data Protection Act 1998). Incorrect entries could adversely affect the client's care, and confuse other professionals. They also reduce your credibility as a competent clinician, especially if your notes are required as evidence in a court of law.

In order to ensure accuracy it may be necessary to correct errors in a record. Strike these through with a single line so that the original entry is not erased or made illegible. This is crucial if litigation arises as it may impede a case or raise suspicions if information has been erased. Always date and at the very least initial your correction.

◊  Relevant

Under the Data Protection Act (1998) only data that is relevant for the purpose for which it was obtained must be kept. Be clear about why you record certain information. Sometimes details are recorded that are not relevant to the care of the client. This may be something the health professional records out of habit or may be an historical feature of a particular department's style of note-keeping. For example, it is often noted about women being single parents. Would you be able to justify recording this information in your own health care context?

◊  Complete

A complete record will contain information sufficient for its purpose without the need for the reader to refer to other sources. It should contain all the information the reader requires to reach the same conclusions as the health professional who wrote it. The Data Protection Act (1998) also requires that personal data obtained, processed and stored is adequate for its purpose.

◊  Accessible

There is no point in having well-executed clinical records if these notes are unavailable or take an enormous amount of time to locate. The clinician can help in the process of efficient information management by completing client identification data. Always ensure that the client's name, date of birth and NHS number or other identifying code are written at the top of the recording sheet. This makes it possible to identify to whom the notes refer, even if sheets become detached from the main file.

Prompt recording of a contact ensures that clinical notes are then available for use by other professionals, and contain the most up-to-date information. Each entry in the record must be signed by the clinician and the full name and title written alongside. This makes it much easier to identify who has made the entry.

◊  Objective

The way information is recorded about the client and his or her condition needs to be without prejudice or bias. Test results and clinical examinations are the easiest to write objectively. It is when results or observations require interpretation that judgements may become subjective.

Aim to be as specific and concrete as possible in your recording. Ask yourself questions – why are you recording this piece of information? What is your evidence for making this judgement? Could you justify to the client what you are writing if challenged to do so?

Remember, bias can occur when we make assumptions or hold stereotypes related to gender, race, sexual orientation, age, socio-economic background, occupation, marital status and even the location of the client's home.

◊  Specific

Be precise in what you record. Avoid giving approximations or making generalisations. For example, 'Jamie has about 10 to 20 words in his vocabulary' is more precise than 'Jamie has a small vocabulary'. Or 'Flora had a little walk today' might be more accurately stated as 'Flora walked five steps today unaided'. Statements like 'doing very well in therapy' tell us very little about the client's actual progress in relation to his or her set goals.

◊  Logical

Information is more accessible and comprehensible if it is organised in a logical way. To some extent, the structure of clinical notes is dictated by the theoretical framework used by the clinician. The traditional medical model focuses on the investigation and treatment of the medical problem, whereas a sociological approach places an emphasis on socio-economic background, family support and the functional aspects of the client's condition. These conceptual models provide the health professional with a guide about how to cluster and order information.

However, within these frameworks there will still be a need for the clinician to give some consideration to organising clinical notes into a rational and logical sequence. A general principle is that entries are recorded consecutively, and recording sheets are filed in chronological order. This helps to show the development and progress of care.

◊ Clear

Health records are a means of communication, and they therefore need to be clear and comprehensible to the reader. Increased access to records means that we need to write notes in the anticipation that the reader may be the client – so avoid unnecessary jargon and abbreviations. The emphasis is on *unnecessary*, as the use of abbreviations can increase the speed of writing notes. Some employers allow abbreviations to be used if they are standard amongst the team and a glossary is available if clients wish to access their records. Personal styles of notation are to be avoided.

Another major obstacle to clarity in manual records is illegible handwriting. Sometimes entries in notes are unreadable, which completely defeats the purpose of recording them in the first place. Progress towards computer-held records is one way of dealing with this problem, as typed entries do not present the same challenge in deciphering the message. Copies of clinical notes may be required in order to provide clients with access to their health records, when dealing with a complaint, or by a court of law. Entries written in black ink are more legible than blue or other coloured inks when photocopied.

◊ Timely

Information recorded about a contact with a client must be recorded as near to that event as possible. This is primarily to ensure that the clinician is able to recall the details and record them as accurately as possible. Second, the most up-to-date information is then available to any health professional accessing the health record of the client.

Clinicians must also be aware that evidence for use in court must be from a record that is contemporaneous with the event to which it relates (Quantum Development 2000). The Department of Health recommends recording information as soon as possible after the contact and at least within the same working day. Twenty-four hours is seen as the maximum. Any delay in recording notes may reduce the credibility of the professional in any complaint.

## Summary Points

- Information needs to be accurate, complete, relevant and accessible if it is to be of use to the health professional, whether this is a clinician, manager or administrator.

- Health records are a means of communication and therefore need to be clear and comprehensible to other clinicians and any clients who may want access.

- Health professionals must strive to avoid any bias or prejudice in the way that they record client information.

- Record keeping must be timely.

# 3

# The Legal Framework

This chapter provides a guide to some of the key issues relating to record keeping and the management of health information. It is not meant to be a definitive account, and the reader is advised to refer to the relevant legislation, health service circulars and guidance notes for a full and complete account. Professional bodies and employers also provide standards in relation to health records management.

There are four main issues to be considered in the management of health information:

1. Accountability

2. Use and protection of client information

3. Access to health records

4. Retention of health records.

## 1. Accountability

A health record is a document that contains information about the physical or mental health of an identified individual, which has been made by or on behalf of a health professional in connection with the care of that individual (Data Protection Act 1998). Although the majority of records are paper based (manual records), there are an increasing number of computer-based notes (electronic records). Health information may also be recorded in other ways such as on audio or visual cassette and CD-ROM.

All NHS records are deemed public records under the Public Records Act (1958), and there are various levels of accountability relating to their management. The clinician is responsible for any records he or she creates or uses. However, it is the NHS Trust or health authority that usually has ownership and copyright of these records (NHS Executive 1999). Chief executives and senior managers in these organisations are personally accountable for the quality of the systems for managing records.

What does accountability mean for the clinician?

- Clinicians are responsible for the professional opinions they have written in the health record.

- Health records remain the property of the employing body, so records remain within the organisation and do not move with the health professional.

- Clinicians must make sure that they know, understand and adhere to their employer's guidelines on information management.

- Clinicians must make sure that they know, understand and adhere to the guidelines issued by their professional body on information management.

- Clinicians who are also line managers are responsible for making sure that their staff are adequately trained in information management and adhere to the guidelines.

## 2. Use and protection of client information

A clinician has always had a common-law duty of confidentiality to his or her clients. In addition health records are covered by the Data Protection Act (1998), which stipulates that all processing of data must be fair and lawful within the context of common law. Therefore clinicians, NHS organisations and so on must comply with the common law of confidentiality when processing personal health information. Clinicians also have a duty to uphold their professional ethical code to keep client information confidential.

A review of how the NHS manages and protects client information used for non-clinical purposes was carried out by a committee chaired by Dame Fiona Caldicott. Its report in 1997 made a number of recommendations for improving confidentiality and ensuring that access to personal health data was strictly on a need to know basis. Caldicott guardians have been appointed in all NHS organisations with the remit to oversee the safeguarding of confidentiality. The role is mainly advisory but the guardian may help in the implementation of improvements.

Further support for the protection of personal information comes from 'The Patient's Charter', which states that the client should expect the right to confidentiality at all times:

> to know that everyone working for the NHS is under a legal duty to keep your records confidential. (Department of Health 1995)

In general, personal information provided in confidence may not be used for any other purpose or by anyone else other than that agreed with the provider (Data Protection Act 1998).

Clients must be informed about the different purposes for which information is collected about them and with whom it may be shared (NHS Executive 1996). Information is gathered primarily to plan and deliver optimum health care to the client. However there are a number of other important uses that include ensuring effective health care administration (for example, clinical audit and risk management), teaching and research.

The Department of Health recommends that clients are told how information might be shared before they are asked to provide it. This might be through the use of general information contained in leaflets and specific discussions between the client and the clinician as part of joint care planning.

However, it is recognised that in health care it would be impracticable and unnecessary to obtain the client's specific consent each time information needed to be passed on. Health professionals must be able to respond to the needs of clients promptly. Personal health information needs to be readily available so that the most appropriate and effective care is delivered. Therefore health organisations need to advise clients that their personal information may need to be shared amongst health staff and with associated agencies, in order to plan and co-ordinate care.

The client has a right to refuse permission for information to be passed on (subject to the exceptions detailed below). Clinicians will need to respect the wishes of the client in such cases. However it is important that clients are made aware of the likely implications of this decision for their own health care and the impact on effective management of health services in general.

### Children and young people
There is often some confusion regarding the rights of children and young people with regard to consent and confidentiality when receiving health care.

- Young people aged 16 or 17 years of age have the right to consent to treatment unless there is evidence of a lack of capacity (the Family Law Reform Act 1969). Consequently such young people also have the same rights to confidentiality as adults.

- Children under 16 may be able to consent to treatment if they are deemed to have a sufficient level of maturity, understanding and competence to make that decision. In such cases the child would also have the right to confidentiality. In other cases the person with parental responsibility, who has consented to treatment on behalf of the child, would be involved in decisions about passing on information.

There are certain exceptions to the duty of confidentiality where information may be disclosed. Below are some examples:

- Where there is a statutory requirement to pass on information, for instance notification of communicable disease, the Public Health (Control of Disease) Act 1984, the Mental Health Act (1983), the Prevention of Terrorism Act (1989).

- Where there is a court order for disclosure of information, for instance during legal proceedings in an action for personal injury.

- In child protection cases the interests of the child take precedence (the Children Act 1989). It may therefore be necessary to share information with specific professionals and agencies.

- Where information needs to be released in order to protect the general public. This often relates to the prevention of serious crime but can include such matters as a public health risk.

What does use and protection of information mean for the clinician?

- Clinicians need to safeguard information provided by clients in the course of receiving health care:

  - Manual records
    This means keeping records in a secure place with access only by authorised personnel, and avoiding accidental

disclosure by not leaving written notes unattended or in view of others. Any unwanted paperwork containing personal details about clients must be disposed of using processes that protect confidentiality. This would normally be by shredding or incineration of the records.

- o Data on computer
  Clinicians should not reveal any information that might compromise the security of a computerised records system. For instance, they should not reveal passwords or allow others access to the computer under their identity and password. Care should be taken that computer screens are not left unattended or in view of public areas.

- o Clinicians must only use client-identifiable information when it is absolutely necessary, and must make sure that it is the minimum required for the purpose.

- o Clinicians need to advise clients prior to obtaining or receiving information about how that information will be used and with whom it may be shared.

- o Clinicians need to discuss with clients the choices available to them about disclosure of information.

- o Clinicians must check whether the client wants family and carers informed about progress, and note this on the record. (It is important that notes kept in the home do not compromise the client's confidentiality in this matter. Some information may need to be held on record in the office base.)

- o All decisions about disclosure of information need to be noted in the health record.

- o Information obtained by clinicians for one purpose may not be used for another without the consent of the client. (See above for exceptions to this rule.)

- o Clinicians must submit for approval any research proposals that require access to personal health records to the Local Research Ethics Committee.

- o Clinicians must obtain the specific consent of clients for any research or teaching that would involve them personally.

- Clinicians need to ascertain, when sharing information about clients with other professionals, that they have the same requirements regarding confidentiality (Shaw 2001).

### 3. Access to health records

Clients have had the right to have access to automatically processed health records since the first Data Protection Act in 1984. This has now been replaced by the Data Protection Act (1998), which came into force on 1 March 2000. This Act permits access to all manual and electronic health records regardless of when they were created. It should be noted that this Act also repeals the Access to Health Records Act (1990), except for provisions concerning the deceased. (The 1990 Act gave individuals the right of access to health information processed manually about themselves from 1 November 1991.)

Clinicians need to note the following provisions of the 1998 Data Protection Act:

- The Act covers both manual and electronic health records.
- Most NHS information (except anonymised information) will be covered by the Act.
- The Act permits access to manual records whenever they were made (subject to certain exceptions detailed below).

There are certain circumstances when access may be limited, for example:

1. Information may not be disclosed if it is thought that it might cause serious physical or mental harm to any person (including any health professional).

2. Information about a third party may not be disclosed without their consent (although this does not include health professionals who may have been involved in compiling or contributing to the record).

3. Where there is a statutory restriction on the disclosure of information; for example, the NHS Trusts and Primary Care Trusts (Sexually Transmitted Diseases) Directions 2000, the Human Fertilisation and Embryology (Disclosure of Information) Act of 1992 both place limitations on the disclosure of certain information.

Apart from the client there are a number of other individuals who might have the right of access. These include persons authorised by the client, a representative appointed by a court of law to manage the client's affairs, a legal representative of a deceased person or anyone having a claim arising from that client's death.

Clients not only have the right to access but also, where appropriate, the right to rectification. They may apply either through the courts or the Data Protection Commissioner to have any inaccurate data and opinions based on that data rectified or removed (Data Protection Act 1998).

What does access to health records mean for the clinician?

- Clinicians need to be aware of the client's rights to access.

- Clinicians must familiarise themselves with their employer's policies on responding to requests from clients for access.

- Clinicians may still allow informal access to records if appropriate (subject to their organisational guidelines), and where any third party information is not likely to be compromised. Sharing of health records with the client is recognised as good practice and is one way of involving them in the health care process. Patient-held records are already used in some areas of health care.

- Health records must be written in the anticipation that clients may exercise their right of access.

- Clinicians will be involved in discussions about formal requests for access and whether any limitations might need to be applied.

- Clinicians may need to prepare an extract from the records or be available to discuss information with the client.

## 4. Retention of health records

There are recommended minimum periods of retention for health records. The length of time varies according to the type of record. There are three types of document – primary, secondary and transitory.

Primary documents would include casenote folders, client identification information, admission sheets, referral letters, case history sheets, assessment or examination information, progress notes, operation sheets, nursing careplans, therapy notes, reports and anaesthetic sheets.

Primary documents have to be retained for a legal minimum period (NHS Executive 1999):

- ○ *Maternity records* must be kept for 25 years.

- ○ *Records of children and young persons* need to be kept until the person's 25th birthday (or 26th if they were 17 years old at the conclusion of treatment). In cases where a child has died before they are 18, the records must be retained for eight years after the death.

- ○ *Mental health records* must be kept for 20 years after no further treatment is considered necessary or eight years following the death of the client if the client died whilst still receiving treatment.

- ○ *Clients involved in clinical trials* must have their records kept for 15 years after the conclusion of treatment.

- ○ *Donor records* must be kept for 11 years post-transplantation.

- ○ *All other personal health records* not covered above must be retained for eight years after the completion of treatment. The conclusion of treatment includes all follow-up checks and actions in connection with that treatment.

Recommended minimum retention periods for GP records are similar except for:

- ○ *Records relating to personnel serving in HM Armed Forces or persons serving a prison sentence* are not to be destroyed (NHS Executive 1998).

- ○ *All other records* not covered above must be retained for a period of ten years (NHS Executive 1998).

Secondary documents (for example x-rays and drug sheets) and transitory documents (for example blood pressure charts) are retained for periods of time determined by locally agreed policies.

What does retention of health records mean for the clinician?

- ○ Records, even damaged ones, must be retained for the recommended minimum periods.

- ○ Clinicians should familiarise themselves with the employer's system for managing records of clients where the duty of care has been discharged.

○ Clinicians should acquaint themselves with the recommended periods of retention of health records and other documents. For instance, diaries, annual leave requests and job descriptions are just some of the documents covered by the regulations.

## Summary Points

○ All health records are deemed public records. Health professionals are responsible for the records they create and use, but the NHS Trust or health authority usually has ownership and copyright of these records.

○ All health professionals have a common-law duty of confidentiality and are bound by professional and ethical standards of confidentiality.

○ Clients need to be made aware that information might need to be shared with other health professionals. They should be told about their choice in deciding with whom information may be shared.

○ Any information given for one purpose may not be used (subject to certain exemptions) for another purpose without the consent of the person who provided it.

○ NHS organisations need to maintain good quality systems for the recording, storing and destruction of health records, confidentiality being of paramount importance.

○ The Data Protection Act of 1998 gives clients the right (subject to certain exemptions) of access to automatically and manually processed health records, regardless of when they were created.

○ Health records must be retained for minimum periods of time recommended by the Department of Health.

# 4

# Clinical Skills in Context
## Record Keeping

### Personal health records

Clinicians will be contributing to the personal health records of a variety of clients on a daily basis. These clinical notes are essential for ensuring the delivery of appropriate and effective care. They will contain information on investigations, diagnosis, care and intervention.

A complete record will also include the views of the client and family in addition to those of the health professional. There will be an account of the client's and the family's understanding of and reaction to the presenting problem. It will also give a description of their wishes, responses to and participation in the delivery of care and treatment.

### Record keeping skills

Health professionals are personally accountable for what they have written in health records. With the increase in litigation it is more important than ever that clinicians ensure that records are complete and comprehensive. For instance, records are one way that competent practice may be demonstrated when a client has complained (Fisher 2001). Record keeping skills must therefore be seen as an essential clinical skill.

The ability to record, interpret and disseminate written information about a client, like any other clinical skill, is essential. Record keeping skills must:

- form a fundamental component of pre-qualification training
- be considered part of professional development and undergo the same scrutiny as other clinical skills and knowledge

- be considered one of the essential elements of clinical practice and therefore be regularly reviewed by the reflective practitioner

- be included in clinical audit so that standards of recording are not only maintained but also areas for improvement are identified

- be regularly updated to take into account the rapid changes in information management and the introduction of new technologies.

Advice is offered about record keeping by various professional bodies, and is often set down as standards to which members are expected to adhere.

Employers also have a statutory duty under the Health Act (1999) to monitor and improve the quality of health care. This would include auditing the standard of record keeping on a regular basis to ensure that the quality of information management is maintained (Dimond 2000).

It is therefore essential that clinicians familiarise themselves with the requirements of both the association representing their particular discipline and their employers.

### When do I need to record?

It is recognised as good practice to record every contact with the client. This includes indirect as well as direct contacts.

A direct contact means any face-to-face interaction with the client, such as carrying out a test or providing treatment.

An indirect contact relates to any actions you carry out that are related to meeting the needs of a specific client. Your contact is *about* the client, but not necessarily *with* the client. This might be liaison, advising family and carers or attending meetings such as case conferences. It would also include recording indirect contacts initiated by other professionals, for example receiving a telephone call regarding one of your clients.

It may be the case that not all of your planned contacts occur, for example clients may fail to attend. Always record the reasons why a planned contact has not taken place. The same rule applies to indirect contacts. For example, make a note of any attempts to liaise with other professionals even if you are unable to get in touch with them. This provides evidence of not only your intended actions for that client, but also the reasons why these may not have been fulfilled.

*How is writing, done in my field?*

Always date and sign each entry regarding a contact. It is also advisable to record the time, especially if you make a series of direct or indirect contacts with a specific client on the same day. This helps to show the development of events, often a critical issue in litigation cases.

Give the name of the location where the client was seen, for example on a home visit, as an out-patient or in the community clinic. Include the name of the hospital or clinic.

*What do I need to record?*

A complete health record will provide the reader with all the information required to reach the same conclusions as the health professional who wrote the notes. There should be no need to refer to other sources.

The type and amount of information noted would be determined by the clinical need of the client, and the context in which the client is seen. For example, documenting an acute episode would vary from the on-going documentation required in a long-stay care facility.

The position of the client along the care pathway will also have a bearing on deciding the content of notes. The main stages in the health care process are:

- referral
- initial assessment
- intervention (including on-going evaluation)
- discharge
- post-discharge.

The following sections offer guidance on the type of information to record at each stage of the care pathway. However, each clinician is reminded to refer to the standards and practices set down by his or her employing organisation and his or her professional body.

### Setting up a personal health record

A personal health record is set up for the client either when a referral is received by the service or at the first contact with the client. The Audit Commission (1995), in a study of hospital records, found that there was no common approach to how these records were organised. They suggested that notes have a clear structure that is agreed with the users – that is, the health professionals and the administrative staff.

A basic principle for any health record is to ensure that information is filed chronologically. This will help users in identifying the current episode and the most recent entry. Arranging data into specific sections like assessments, treatment and so on may also help the reader to quickly locate the relevant information.

Every clinician has a responsibility to check, update and maintain the client records they are using.

### Identification details

Each health record must contain the personal details that will enable the identification of the client to whom the information pertains. This will usually include the client's:

- names (at least the first and the last name)
- title (Mr/Miss/Mrs/Dr)
- form of address preferred by the client (for example, first name or title with last name)
- address
- telephone number
- date of birth
- identification number (for example NHS number, social security number, *number* issued by health provider).

Other relevant information would include:

- the name and address of the next of kin/carer/guardian
- preferred form of address for the next of kin/carer/guardian
- name and address of the client's general practitioner
- details of other professionals in regular contact with the client.

### Referral stage

One of the key pieces of information to note in the health record is the reason why the client is being seen by your service. It is often the case that clients are referred by another health professional or an associated agency such as social services. In some cases there may be no referring agent, for instance clients who self-refer, or emergency admissions to accident and emergency. You will therefore need to record the circumstances or incident that has prompted the client's attendance.

Part of the record at this point in the process will include the client's account of the reason for his or her contact with your service. In some cases it may be appropriate to also make a note about the attitude of the client or the family towards the referral. For example, parents may disagree that an appointment with the clinical psychologist is necessary, but still attend the appointment at the behest of the child's school.

A complete record at the referral stage in the care process will show:

- the name and position of the referrer
- the date of the referral
- the reason for the referral.

Key documents to be kept on file:

- referral letters/admission forms
- reports accompanying referral.

### Initial assessment

Assessment is a process that will involve gathering information through interview, observation, clinical investigations and objective and behavioural tests. The type of information collected will relate to the theoretical approach of the record's user (Pagano and Ragan 1992) – so the assessment process of a medic will differ from that of a nurse, and both will differ from that of a therapist.

It is essential that, whenever possible, consent is obtained from the client before assessment is initiated. This consent must be informed and the clinician has the responsibility to make sure that the client understands the nature of any assessment procedures, their purpose and any risks. Consent, whether it is given verbally, in writing or by implication, must be recorded in the notes. See the section in this chapter on 'Writing a Careplan' for a fuller discussion on recording consent and communicating risk.

In general, the type of client data that is collected in assessment will include information about:

- physical signs, symptoms and behaviours that indicate the client's current health status
- current health care (for example information on medication, other illnesses)

- o  psychological factors (for example mood and client's response to the problem)
- o  psychosocial factors (for example culture, religion)
- o  predisposing factors to the problem
- o  cognitive skills (for example memory, language skills)
- o  environment (for example type of housing or support from family)
- o  lifestyle (for example habits, diet and exercise)
- o  daily living pattern (for example working, retired or looking after young children)
- o  self-care abilities
- o  risk factors (for example is the client prone to falls? Is there a family history of a similar condition? Allergies?).

In children you will also want to include information about developmental and behavioural patterns (Cohen 1983).

Client data is used by the clinician:

- o  to identify the health problem, formulate a diagnosis and determine the likely prognosis
- o  to determine the need for further in-depth assessment or referral to other professionals
- o  to provide a baseline measure for evaluating progress
- o  to establish the need for intervention and prioritise individual clients within the general caseload
- o  to help plan intervention and set realistic outcomes
- o  to help plan for discharge.
- ◊  To identify the health problem, formulate a diagnosis and determine the likely prognosis.

Taking a case history is an essential first step in collecting relevant client data. Information is usually provided directly by the client, but in some circumstances another may give it, such as a parent or friend. In the latter case, always record the name and relationship of the informant to the client.

Write a description of the problem using the client's own words. Note the way in which it first became apparent to him or her and the development of the problem. The onset and sequence of symptoms need to be dated as accurately as possible. Establish whether the problem has changed in character or severity, and note any circumstances that are associated with these changes – also, what does it mean for the client, impact on lifestyle, degree of pain and so on.

The information provided in the case history will be supported by your clinical observations, and by objective or behavioural tests that help to describe and quantify the presenting problem. This information is the evidence on which your clinical decision making is based and must be clearly recorded in the client's notes.

A set of complete notes will also have a record of planned assessments that were abandoned or postponed. Give the reasons for this: for example, the client was too tired to complete a psychological test, or the client was unable to tolerate a procedure due to the pain. Record how you plan to follow this up: for example, date for a follow-up appointment or referral for an alternative procedure.

Once sufficient information has been collected then the clinician is in a position to interpret the data. A professional judgement can be made about the diagnosis by labelling either a health problem or the client's needs. Once this is known, an opinion regarding the likely prognosis is possible about both the health of the client and the outcome of intervention. These clinical decisions may be noted as bullet points at the end of your entry in the record. Remember to note your discussions with the client regarding the findings of the assessment and your agreed actions.

◊ To determine the need for further in-depth assessment or referral to other professionals.

Some clients may need further assessment or referral to other services. Your notes need to show that you have identified this need and have action planned for this. The reason for any referral needs to be clearly recorded along with the client's views upon it and obviously their agreement to it.

Record information about:

- ○ Referrals to other agencies. (Keep copies of letters or referral forms on file.)

- ○ Liaison with other professionals. This will include attempts to make contact with other professionals even if they were unsuccessful. This will show when and how you have attempted to act upon the information you have gained about the client's clinical need.

○ Details of any further assessments with a plan for when and how these will be carried out.

◊ To provide a baseline measure for evaluating progress.

Your assessment will provide detailed information on the current health status of the client. This will then form a benchmark against which change, whether this is progress or deterioration, can be measured. Future users of the personal health record must be clear about:

○ your actions (assessments, investigations and so on) along with the date

○ the results

○ your interpretation of these results

○ your clinical decisions based on that interpretation

○ your actions based on those decisions

○ your recommendations for future management.

This information will help focus subsequent examinations and investigations, thus facilitating continuity of care. It also helps prevent needless repetition of investigations.

◊ To establish the need for intervention and prioritise clinical need.

Your assessment will help you make decisions about whether a client requires intervention and the degree of urgency about when this will happen. These decisions will be based on your judgement of the client's clinical needs and whether resources (staff, drugs, equipment and so on) are available to meet them. You will also want to note information about the client's likely compliance and potential for change.

Information that will help in your decision making includes:

○ the impact of the problem on the client's lifestyle and quality of life (for children, this would include the impact of the problem on development, socialisation and education)

○ the client's risk of the problem increasing or worsening

○ the client's expectations

- ○ the client's physical and psychological response to any previous treatment
- ○ the client's likely compliance
- ○ the client's readiness for intervention (this will depend on the psychological, physical, psychosocial, behavioural and developmental status of the client).

◊ To help plan intervention and set realistic outcomes.

Assessment must be both comprehensive and complete in order to plan appropriate and effective intervention. Information that will help you make judgements about the predicted or likely outcome of any intervention includes:

- ○ any factors in the client or the client's environment that may hinder change or perpetuate the problem (these may need to be addressed prior to or as part of any planned intervention)
- ○ factors indicating the potential for change:
  - ○ the client's likely compliance (including motivation)
  - ○ factors that might impact on the client's ability to achieve outcomes, for example age, cognitive, sensory and educational abilities
  - ○ the support available to the client in achieving outcomes
  - ○ the client's previous responses to intervention (What has worked before? What problems have occurred?)
  - ○ the limitations placed on the client's lifestyle and quality of life by their health problem
- ○ the client's health education needs.

◊ To help plan for discharge.

Record any information relevant to the preparation for discharge. The amount of information gathered at this stage will depend on the nature and extent of your contact with the client. Useful information would include:

- ○ the client's likely continuing health needs after your duty of care is completed
- ○ the client's access to on-going health care after your duty of care is completed

    o   the client's support network, for example does the client live
        alone?

This will give some indication of the client's likely needs and the available
support after discharge.

### Summaries

A large amount of information is often gathered at the assessment stage.
Writing a summary helps the clinician in communicating the key findings
in a succinct manner that is easily accessed by future users of the personal
health record. A summary will include statements about diagnosis (prognosis if appropriate), actions and recommendations.

    A complete record at the assessment stage in the care process will
show:

- the details of any relevant history
- the details of assessments administered and examinations or
  investigations carried out, along with the date these were
  performed
- the results of these tests, investigations and procedures
- diagnosis (and prognosis where applicable)
- actions arising out of the assessment (for example referral
  elsewhere, advice, waiting list for treatment)
- identification of the type and extent of clinical intervention
- prioritisation information
- plans for future management that include a date for review
- the client's views and concerns regarding the above
  information
- the name and position of the clinician who evaluated the
  client.

Key documents to be kept on file at the assessment stage:

- a case history form or admission sheet
- forms or charts used in tests, investigations or procedures
- consent forms signed by the client giving permission for
  investigations

❑ a copy of any reports or letters circulated about the initial assessment

❑ copies of referral letters to other agencies or health professionals

❑ copies of any information provided by the client or family.

## Intervention

A primary function of the personal health record is to describe the actions taken to meet the needs of the client. You need to show that your care for the client was planned, regularly monitored and the outcome evaluated. Your notes will also include evidence of the client's involvement and agreement with your proposed plan of care (Moody 2001).

### *Planning intervention*

The purpose of any intervention is to achieve a positive effect on the health status of the client. This might be in their physiological, psychological, behavioural, social or developmental function.

The main aims of intervention are:

○ to anticipate and reduce the risk of any deterioration in health status or function

○ to ameliorate problems and restore premorbid or developmentally appropriate levels of functioning

○ to maximise the client's level of functioning within the limits imposed by their current health status

○ to preserve the current level of health status or functioning

○ to prevent or delay deterioration in the client's health status or level of functioning

○ to increase the client's knowledge and skills in coping with the health problem

○ to support the client and the client's significant others in accepting and coping with the client's health status or level of functioning

○ to alleviate the psychological or physiological discomfort or distress of the client.

Before commencing intervention you will have formed a plan of action based on your reason for care, which needs to be noted in the client's personal health record. There are various ways of recording this information. You may write it directly into the progress notes of the client's personal health record, or you may be required to complete a careplan. The latter is often a standardised, pre-prepared document.

Care pathways (or clinical pathways) are a recent initiative to develop a standardised multidisciplinary careplan that describes key interventions along a timeline. They include expected outcomes and outline the main stages in the clinical management of the client. Care Pathways are being developed for specific procedures and client groups.

However, as a clinician you might also be involved in creating an individualised plan for the client, either because there is no documented pathway or the specific needs of the client require an individual management plan.

Careplans describe:

- your intended actions for the client
- your objectives (what the actions will achieve)
- the timeframe.

Careplans are evidence that the care for the client was planned and that there was a clear rationale to support the clinical decision making. They also provide a written record to which other health staff are able to refer thus ensuring continuity of care. Careplans are also a way of sharing information with the client.

## Writing a careplan

Part of writing a careplan is selecting the most appropriate objectives for your specific client.

Remember to:

◊ Set objectives *with* the client and not *for* the client
  The client who participates in setting his or her own goals is more likely to understand and be committed to the care process. (See the discussion below about recording consent to treatment.)

◊ Prioritise
  Information from assessment will help you make decisions about priorities for the individual client, which will be set against the needs identified in your overall caseload. In some cases the priorities might be obvious, for example acute clinical need must be addressed first. However, much of your decision making will

involve establishing what the priorities are for the client. This will often involve negotiation and compromise by both you and the client.

◊ Make the goals realistic

Your choice of goals will be influenced by:

- ○ Your assessment of the client's needs.

- ○ Your clinical experience – what you know has worked before with other clients and how long it took to achieve it.

- ○ Evidence based practice – research will help you select appropriate and efficacious treatment. Make use of care pathways (or clinical pathways) whenever possible. They have been developed by multidisciplinary experts using sound scientific evidence.

- ○ Individual differences between clients. These factors will mean that the type, amount and length of intervention will vary between clients. For example, an elderly client may need a longer timescale.

- ○ The environment – what are the opportunities and limitations arising from the care environment, home or family situation? For example, the development of independent living skills may be difficult in a hospital setting where meals and so on are provided.

- ○ The timescale – what is your estimate of the time needed to achieve the goal? What amount of time is available to work with the client?

Remember that goals set in conjunction with the client are more likely to be something that he or she feels is achievable.

◊ Set your objectives in conjunction with other team members
Check that your objectives link in with those set by other members of the health team or other relevant professionals. This will help avoid any duplication and ensure that goals complement rather than contradict each other. Again care pathways (or clinical pathways) provide a multidisciplinary perspective on the management of the client. The pathway is a shared careplan.

◊ Consider organisational guidelines

Write objectives that comply with organisational guidelines. For example, an objective about a client self-administering medication will be contraindicated in a setting where organisational or professional guidelines prohibit this.

◊ Evaluate risk

A planned objective must not put the client or others at unacceptable risk. This is partly an unacceptable risk when compared with recognised best practice, and also what the individual client deems an unacceptable risk. Clients will vary in risk acceptance, and this will influence their decision making about treatment regimes. Therefore it must be made clear to the client about any likely risks or negative outcomes arising from intervention, for example the side effects of a specific drug regime. Careful explanation of these risks is required if clients are to make informed choices about their treatment. These choices will depend on the client understanding and accepting potential and actual risk. Such a discussion needs to be recorded in the notes in order to provide the clinician with protection from any future litigation.

### Recording clients' decisions regarding consent to treatment

It is essential that whenever possible, consent is obtained from the client before the start of treatment. Consent, whether it is given verbally, in writing or by implication, must be recorded in the notes. Your records also need to show not only that the client consented but also that he or she was capable of making this decision. The client must have sufficient information to consider the benefits and the risks of the proposed treatment in order to make a decision (Rodgers 2000). Consent must be informed.

It is the clinician's responsibility to make sure that the client understands:

  ○ the nature of any procedures

  ○ the likely positive and negative outcomes

  ○ the risks.

Part of this explanation might include the option to 'do nothing' and the associated benefits and/or risks. A record of the information given to the client is therefore an important part of the health record and might become a vital factor if litigation arises.

There are various ways of noting the decision to consent:

○ A narrative account is written directly into the progress notes.

○ The client agrees and signs a careplan, which includes consent to treatment. One copy is kept on file, and one copy is kept by the client.[1]

○ Standardised pre-prepared consent forms are signed by the client and are kept on file. (Written consent forms are required in certain circumstances, for example under the Abortion Act 1967.) Check your organisational guidelines regarding written consent.

○ The client is involved in recording his or her progress in treatment (evidence of implied consent).[1]

Regardless of which method you choose you will need to be specific about the actions to which the client is consenting. This will also include a reference to the period of time to which the consent applies.

### Children and young people

Consent for children under the age of 16 is most likely to be given by an adult with parental responsibility, although, in some cases, it may be the child who gives consent to treatment (see 'Use and Protection of Information' in Chapter 3). The above advice on providing information applies equally to this client group. The clinician must ensure that sufficient information is given to the adult or child giving consent to treatment. Again, discussions about consent must be clearly recorded in the notes.

### Refusal of treatment

A refusal by the client of proposed treatment needs to be noted. This applies whether it is the whole or only parts of the treatment with which the client refuses to proceed. Record the reasons for refusal using the client's words wherever possible, and detail your advice to the client on the possible risks or negative outcomes of his or her decision. This will provide evidence to help protect the clinician against any future litigation for negligence. It will also provide useful information for other health professionals on the client's attitudes, beliefs and wishes.

Extraordinary circumstances, such as clients with 'living wills' or those who have religious objections to certain medical procedures such as blood transfusions, require special attention to record keeping. It is important to check organisational and professional guidelines on procedures, which should include directions about record keeping.

*Difficulties in obtaining consent*

In some cases there may be difficulties or barriers to communicating the necessary information to clients. Examples might include clients with a different language from the clinician, clients with a communication disability following a stroke or clients with a hearing loss. It may be necessary to use interpreters or advocates to help communicate information effectively about treatment options. Whatever method is used it is important that the way in which the client's consent was obtained is clearly recorded.

*Clients who are not competent to consent*

In certain circumstances it may not be possible to obtain consent from the client prior to giving treatment, for example an unconscious client in accident and emergency. The reason for not obtaining consent must always be recorded, along with information about how a client was deemed to be incompetent to give consent. This is particularly important in the case of clients with a mental health problem, and special forms are available for these situations (NHS Executive 1990).

**Writing your objectives**

Use the following guidelines to help you set clear, realistic and measurable goals for your client.

◊ Be client focused
   Write goals that focus on what you expect the client to achieve, and not on your actions as the clinician or on the type of intervention.

For example:

'To advise client on a gluten-free diet.'

✕ This is about the clinician's actions.

'Client to state foods to avoid for a gluten-free diet.'

✓ The focus is on the actions of the client.

◊ Use positive statements
King *et al.* (1983) suggest using positive terms instead of words like 'if' or 'try' (words that are associated with the possibility of failure). Such choices of language are important when careplans are being set with the client.

For example:
   ✗ Client to try to walk for 10 minutes a day.
   ✓ Client to walk for 10 minutes a day.

◊ Focus on the desired behaviour rather than the undesired one
Again, an important consideration when careplans are shared with the client.

For example:
   ✗ Client to reduce stammering on telephone.
   ✓ Client to use fluent speech on telephone.

◊ Make objectives measurable
Making an objective measurable provides you with a systematic way of evaluating the result or outcome of your intervention. Use specific statements in your objectives that contain information about quantifiable behaviours to be observed in the client.

Springhouse (1998) suggests that such statements will include the following three key components:

  ◦ an observable behaviour

  ◦ a measure of that behaviour

  ◦ the condition under which that behaviour will occur.

◊ An observable behaviour
A behaviour must be observable in order that you can detect change versus no change. Behaviours may be classified as:

  ◦ a physical response (for example blood pressure)

  ◦ a psychological response (for example mood)

  ◦ a skill (for example speech)

  ◦ a personal habit (for example smoking)

  ◦ a social response (for example eye-contact).

  ◦ A measure of that behaviour

You need to have some idea about how you will quantify the behaviour. The following questions will help you find suitable measures:

- How often will it occur (frequency)?
- When will it occur?
- How long will it last for (length)?
- Are there any limits on the behaviour (extent or range)?
- The condition under which that behaviour will occur.

Be specific about under what conditions the behaviour will occur. For example, 'feeding self' – is it aided or unaided by the nurse? Examples of measurable objectives are:
'weight loss of 7 kg at a rate of 1 kg a week'

- behaviour = weight loss
- measure = 7 kg
- condition = 1 kg per week.

'Walking with the assistance of a zimmer frame from his bed to the toilet twice daily'

- behaviour = walking
- measure = from bed to toilet twice daily
- condition = assistance of zimmer frame.

'Reports an increase in skin comfort following application of hydromol emollient cream to eczema from 5 to 9 on a scale of 1 to 10'

- behaviour = reports an increase in skin comfort
- measure = from 5 to 9 on a scale of 1 to 10
- condition = application of hydromol emollient cream to eczema.

'Name the colours (red, blue, yellow, green) with 100% consistency in spontaneous speech'

- behaviour = naming colours
- measure = 100% consistency
- condition = spontaneous speech.

◊ Set a timescale

State when you expect the goals for the client to be achieved.
may not be the same as the review date for the careplan, as g
achieved at different points along the timeline. Make the time
tic. (See 'Make the goals realistic' above.)

**Writing interventions**

Interventions are the actions required to meet the objectives set for the individual client, for example administering care, providing therapy, giving
medication or carrying out a procedure.

Often the clinician will be acting autonomously in choosing and implementing interventions. Selecting the most appropriate action will be
tempered by:

- the client characteristics
- the available resources (both staff and equipment)
- the available skill base (are the appropriately qualified staff
  available?)
- the evidence base
- the guidelines set by your organisation and profession
  (interventions must not contravene standards).

In some circumstances, one health professional may be carrying out interventions prescribed by another. For instance, a district nurse may need to
provide treatment set by the general practitioner. In these circumstances, or
where more than one health professional is implementing the careplan, it
is necessary to detail the interventions.

When writing interventions:

- Be specific.
- Be clear.
- Be realistic.

A good description will provide the reader with information about:

- the specific action
- the procedure for implementing that action (examples would
  be: stating the route for administering medication, the length
  of time to exercise a client's limb or the use of a mirror to aid
  speech exercises)
- when or how often to carry out the action.

Interventions may be written in the progress notes, on the careplan or on standardised forms pre-prepared for this purpose. Whatever the method of recording, it should be clear to which objective the intervention relates and how.

Any unusual or special interventions must be supported by a written record as to why these were necessary.

**Implementation of the careplan**

A record of your contacts with the client during intervention will provide evidence of the quality and quantity of care delivered. This is often referred to as progress notes. It will enable you to share information with colleagues, as well as providing a way of evaluating the outcomes of your actions.

You will need to record the following.

1.  The actions taken to meet the client's needs – both planned and unplanned

    Planned actions are those that relate to the goals stated on the client's careplan. Your entries will make clear:

    o   what was done

    o   how it was done

    o   when it was done

    o   who did it.

    For example, when giving medication the following details are important:

    o   the name of the medication

    o   the dose administered

     = what?

    o   the administration route (oral, intravenous)

    o   the site of administration (for example left arm)

     = how?

    o   date and time administered to the client

     = when?

○ name and signature of clinician

= who?

Unplanned actions might include responding to an emergency situation or a routine but unexpected response from the client during treatment. In these cases you will need to record additional information about the circumstances that prompted your actions.

Write an explanation for any care that it has not been possible to carry out.

2.  The client's response to your actions or to your interventions

Record responses that are indicative of progress, deterioration or no change. This will help form part of your on-going evaluation of the client's progress in relation to the stated goals of intervention. Your observations may lead you to change your original careplan, which must be seen as a dynamic document that is open to modification rather than a static record.

Record any unusual or potentially dangerous events (Pagano and Ragan 1992), for example a fall or self-harming. Check your organisational guidelines on how to record such incidents. There are usually standardised, pre-prepared incident forms designed specifically for this purpose.

3.  Note your observations of the client's general condition

Record any change in symptoms and your actions in response to this.

4.  Note the comments of the client and his or her significant others

Make a note of any discussions with the client and family about progress, intervention and the health problem. Again, record any actions that might arise in response to this.

A summary is often useful when the notes are lengthy or there are several entries during a shift. This enables other staff to quickly assess the current status of the client.

## Evaluation

Although evaluation must be an on-going process throughout intervention, each careplan must also include a review date. This will be the date when you expect the client to have achieved the goals set in his or her careplan. Checking whether the planned outcomes were achieved or not is one way of judging the effectiveness of your intervention.

Note whether each outcome was:

- achieved
- partially achieved
- not achieved.

Record any reasons why an outcome may not have been achieved. Reasons might be:

- Planned goals were unrealistic or inappropriate.
- Non-compliance (for example client not taking medication or failing to comply with a therapy regime).
- Client's progress slower than expected and outcome only partially achieved.
- Change in client's needs (for example a sudden and unexpected deterioration).

Good practice emphasises the involvement of the client and his or her significant others in evaluating outcomes. Make a note of any comments.

Evaluation completes the three parts of the intervention stage:

- planning the careplan
- implementing the careplan
- evaluating the careplan.

A complete record at the intervention stage of the care process will show:

- the client's consent to treatment
- how your intervention was planned
- the actions you have taken to meet the needs of the client
- the reasons or rationale for your actions
- the reasons why any planned actions did not take place
- the client's progress in relation to the stated goals of intervention
- the quantity and quality of the care you have delivered
- that you have fulfilled your duty of care.

Key documents to be kept on file:

- ❑ careplan(s)
- ❑ consent forms for treatment, therapy or surgery

- ❑ progress records
- ❑ incident forms.

## Discharge

Discharge signals the end of the client's episode or episodes of care. The information you record in the notes at this final stage will help to demonstrate the rationale underpinning your decision to close the case.

This would include:

- ○ the results of any assessments, tests or investigations
- ○ the client's progress in relation to the stated goals of intervention
- ○ the client's ability to manage his or her on-going care needs
- ○ the wishes, views and opinions of the client, his or her family and any other significant person.

Your clinical judgement to discharge will be based on all of the above information. Record and date your decision giving your reasons for discharge.

The main reasons for discharge are:

- ○ No intervention is indicated.
- ○ Care of the client is transferred to other services.
- ○ Intervention is no longer required as outcomes are achieved.
- ○ Intervention is no longer appropriate.
- ○ Client declines intervention (always document any voluntary discharge against the advice of the health professional).
- ○ Client has died.

Your notes are also important evidence that the discharge was planned, and that steps were taken to ensure continuity of care for the client. Record the actions you have taken in preparing the client for discharge. This might include:

- ○ enquiries to other agencies regarding support for the client on discharge
- ○ informing relevant agencies regarding the client's on-going needs

- making referrals to other services
- discussions with the client, family and carers.

The referrer, general practitioner and any other key agencies involved with the client will need to know that your involvement is now completed. In cases where the client has died, the clinician may also have personal responsibility to notify colleagues of the death.

Part of discharge will be helping the client and his or her family understand when and at what point your responsibility ends (NHS Training Division 1994). Risk increases if the client is not fully informed, as confusions may arise if further support is needed in the future. The client needs to know:

- the professional or service responsible for any on-going health needs
- the circumstances that would initiate a re-referral to your service
- the route for such a re-referral.

Make a record of not only what discharge information was given to the client but also the views of the client and his or her family about the decision to discharge.

Clients may require directions about medication, self-administered health care or therapy regimes for use post-discharge. Provide such instructions in writing whenever possible. This decreases the chance of error, and reduces the record keeping load as copies of the information can be easily filed in the notes.

Be specific when giving clients information about medication. A medication instruction sheet would have the following:

- client identification data
- name of the medication
- dosage
- when to take it
- how often to take it
- how to take it (for example after a meal with water)
- date of the instruction
- signature (and name in full) with position of prescriber.

Always note any expression of non-compliance regarding discharge instructions, and your actions in response to this.

Much of the above information can be summarised in a discharge report. That can be circulated to the relevant parties and a copy kept on file. (See Chapter 5 on 'Letters and Reports' for the key content of discharge reports.)

A complete record at the discharge stage in the care process will show:

- ○ the date of the decision to discharge
- ○ the reason for discharge
- ○ the clinician or team of clinicians who made the decision
- ○ the views of the client and the client's family and/or significant others
- ○ that discharge was planned
- ○ that continuity of care was planned and appropriate action taken to assist the process
- ○ that risk was assessed and managed.

Key documents to be kept on file:

- ❑ results of assessments and investigations relating to the discharge decision
- ❑ copies of referrals to other services
- ❑ copy of discharge instruction sheets given to clients including directions about medication, self-administered health care or therapy regimes
- ❑ discharge reports.

### Post-discharge

The health records of clients who have been discharged must be retained for the recommended period of time. (See Chapter 3 under 'Retention of Health Records'.) The clinician must comply with organisational guidelines on preparing records for storage. This will include carrying out administrative procedures to record that the notes are in discharge, thereby ensuring easy access to them in the future.

**Action Points**

1. Work with a colleague and audit a sample of each other's clinical notes. Discuss each other's strengths in record keeping. Are there any areas where you are consistent in not meeting the standards? Set yourself a goal to develop these areas. Plan to re-audit your notes within a set timeframe. Have you managed to maintain and improve your record keeping skills?

**Notes**

1     Options that involve clients actively in record keeping are likely to increase their motivation and understanding of the care process.

| | Actions | Record | Keep on file |
|---|---|---|---|
| **Referral/first contact** | * Set up personal health record | * Client identification details<br>* Reason for and date of referral or attendance<br>* Name and position of the referrer | * Referral form or letter/admission slip<br>* Accompanying reports |
| **Initial assessment** | * Evaluate clinical need | * A case history<br>* Client's views about the problem<br>* Clinical observations<br><br>* Tests, investigations and procedures<br>* Interpretation<br>* Diagnosis/prognosis<br>* Actions/recommendations | * Case history form or admission sheet<br><br>* Consent forms for specific investigations<br>* Forms or charts used in tests, investigations or procedures |
| | * Communication about assessment<br>* Refer on as appropriate | * Client's concerns and views on the assessment and outcome | * A copy of reports or letters circulated about the assessment<br>* Copies of referral letters to other professionals |
| **Intervention** | * Set careplan | * Record objectives<br>* Record client's views about careplan | * Consent forms for treatment, therapy or surgery<br>* Careplan |

*Figure 4.1: Summary of record keeping at key stages in the care process*

| | Actions | Record | Keep on file |
|---|---|---|---|
| | * Implement careplan | * Record interventions<br>* Record client's responses | * Progress records |
| | * Evaluate careplan | * Record outcomes<br>* Record clinical decision making | |
| **Discharge** | * Re-evaluation of clinical need | * Results of investigations, tests or procedures<br>* Treatment outcomes<br>* Assessment of the client's ability to manage on-going care needs | * Results of assessments relating to discharge decision |
| | * Preparation for discharge | * Liaison with other agencies<br>* Views of the client and client's family or significant others<br>* Advice/instructions to client and family/carers | * Copies of referrals to other services<br>* Copy of discharge instruction sheets |
| | * Discharge | * Date and reason for the discharge<br>* Name and status of the clinician who made the decision | |
| | * Communication of closure intentions | * Discussion with client/referrer/other professionals about closure intentions | * Discharge report |
| **Post-discharge** | * Retention of records for recommended minimum period of time | * Complete administration procedures relating to storage and future retrieval of records | * File record in secure storage |

*Figure 4.1 cont'd*

# 5

# Letters and Reports

Letters and reports about the care and management of clients are an essential form of communication within the health service. This chapter reviews how to plan, structure and present such correspondence.

## Letters

There are two types of letter – formal and informal. The two are distinguished from each other by different styles, presentation and tone.

Formal letters refer to correspondence that has an official or business function. They are printed or typed on headed paper using a conventional style of composition. The manner of address is formal rather than personal, so the preferred title and last name of the recipient is used to start the letter. They are signed off with the name, position, title and qualifications of the letter writer.

Informal letters are written using a more conversational tone and are sent between two people who know each other. The usual form of address in these letters is by the first name.

Letters are only one of the means of communication available to the health professional; however, they have certain advantages over other methods.

Choose a letter if you want to:

- present complex information and elaborate on ideas
- have time to organise your thoughts and review your intended message
- have a confidential means to convey information

- ○ indicate to the recipient the seriousness of the matter under discussion.

Sometimes a letter is not always the most appropriate or most sensitive choice of communication.

| *If your message:* | *Consider using:* |
| --- | --- |
| is urgent | e-mail, fax, telephone |
| is an apology | telephone, face-to-face contact |
| requires explanation | face-to-face contact, telephone |
| is informal, brief or a reminder | e-mail, memo |
| requires discussion or exchange of ideas or involves decision making | meeting, video or telephone conferencing. |

### Structure of letters

Letters consist of:

- ○ a greeting
- ○ an introduction
- ○ the main body
- ○ the conclusion
- ○ a closing sentence
- ○ a signature.

*Greetings*

The way in which you address the recipient will depend on whether you are writing a formal or informal letter. In certain circumstances a more general term like 'client' or 'parent' may be permissible in letters sent *en masse* or if you are unable to verify the recipient's name.

*Introduction*

The first paragraph will state clearly the reason or purpose for writing.

The following examples show how the use of some pertinent details (including the date) helps the writer indicate the topic or subject of the message to the reader.

In response to a letter or other type of contact – 'Thank you for your letter dated ... regarding ...' or 'Thank you for your phone call on the ... I am sorry I was not available to speak to you personally'; 'I am writing to you regarding your enquiry on the ... about the waiting list for day surgery.'

To make an enquiry – 'I am writing to you regarding the shortage of car parking at Ginsbury Health Centre. I would like to find out whether it would be possible to install a barrier that will restrict access to staff members.'

Some letters start using a traditional format. For example, referral letters usually start with a sentence like: '*Thank you for seeing* this elderly gentleman who has been complaining of chest pains for the last three days.'

### The main body

This contains the main message of the letter along with any supporting details or information.

### Conclusion

The content of the conclusion will vary according to the purpose of the letter. It may include a summary, recommendations, request for action or a statement of what is expected from the recipient.

### Closing sentence

A letter is usually brought to an end by the use of a closing sentence. For example, 'I look forward to hearing from you', 'Please do not hesitate to contact me if you need further information' or 'Thank you for your assistance in this matter.' The addition of phrases such as 'best wishes' or 'kind regards' helps to add a courteous note, particularly in informal letters.

### Signature

Letters must always be signed, as they may be required as evidence in the event of a complaint or litigation. The signature shows that the health professional, or another person authorised to do so in his or her absence, has checked the letter and agreed the content. Formal letters require the signature to be accompanied by the title, position and in some cases the qualifications of the letter writer.

The subscription accompanying the signature will depend on the form of address used in the greeting. A letter starting with 'Dear Sir/Madam' will end with 'Yours faithfully', whereas one starting with the first name, or title and last name, will end with 'Yours sincerely'.

### Layout and format of a letter

Letters are set out according to a standard format. Figure 5.1 is an example of a standard layout.

Remember:

- Keep text well spaced with the left-hand margin aligned with the start of the recipient's address.

- The current style is to have 'open punctuation' (Dobson 1995), where punctuation is kept to a minimum, so avoid using full stops and commas in headings, addresses and dates unless the clarity or meaning is affected by leaving them out.

- Any special messages, like marking the letter 'confidential' or for the attention of a specific person, also need to be marked on the outside of the envelope.

- It is not necessary to repeat headings on any continuation sheets; however, they should be numbered. Mark the bottom of the preceding page with 'cont.'.

- Use 'date as postmark' for large numbers of letters sent out at routine intervals.

- Include identification information on any tear-off slips. Include the name and address of where to return the slip, what it refers to (for example 'diabetes clinic') and any client identification information.

**Heading**
(usually the logo of the organisation)

**Address**
(if not included in
heading)

(check position for window envelopes)

↙

**Name and address of recipient**

↖

(write on separate lines)

↑

(note this starts lower
down the page than
sender's address)

**Date dictated:**

**Date typed:**

**Our ref:** (initials of sender/typist/file number)

**Your ref:** (any reference provided in previous correspondence
from addressee)

(align left-hand margin
with start of address)

↓

*Figure 5.1 Standard format of a letter*

**Dear...**

**Heading**
(subject matter or name, DOB, address of client)

**Introduction**

**Main body**

**Conclusion**

**Closing phrase**

**Yours sincerely/faithfully,**

(note the use of a small 's' and 'f')

**Space for signature**

**Name in full**

(plus preferred form of address/
title, qualifications)

**Position**

(shows the recipient who else has seen
the letter/informs the secretary of the
circulation list)

**Cc** (names of people who will receive a copy)
**Enc.** (detail any enclosures, e.g. maps, timetable)

*Figure 5.1 cont'd*

### Writing a letter

You may be about to write your first clinical letter, either during your clinical practice or as part of an assignment for college. The following section offers some guidance on the four stages in composing such a letter. They are:

1. Preparation
2. Planning
3. Drafting
4. Editing.

### 1. Preparation

#### (a) Decide on your terms of reference

What is your reason for writing the letter? Who is the most appropriate person to receive the letter? What is your timeframe? Who needs a copy of the letter?

An additional question to consider is whether you are the most appropriate person to write the letter. This is essential where situations are litigious. In these cases you may need to refer to a senior colleague or manager before proceeding.

#### (b) Gather your facts

Before starting the letter you need to make sure that you have all the relevant facts and figures. It is important to be accurate and to verify any information. Mistakes in a letter between clinicians may lead to misunderstandings or delays in the assessment and treatment of a client. Remember that your letter, like any other part of a health record, may be used as evidence in a court of law. Any mistakes are likely to reduce your credibility as a competent witness or defendant.

### 2. Planning

You can start to plan your letter once you have established your terms of reference and gathered the necessary information. You will need to select information that is relevant for both the purpose of the letter and the needs of the reader.

*What is the purpose of your letter?*

Think about why you are writing the letter. Is it:

- ° to request information (for example information about previous treatment)

- ° to give information (for example test results)

- ° to request action (for example making a referral)

- ° to confirm an action has taken place (for example a discharge summary)

- ° to organise (for example making an appointment)

- ° to respond (for example replying to a complaint)

- ° to explain requirements (for example explaining procedures for making referrals)?

Always consider your reader during the planning stage:
What does he or she know already?

- ° This will help you to avoid any redundancy in your message.

What does he or she need to know from your letter?

- ° This will help you in selecting relevant information and making your message specific.

What are the reader's expectations of the letter?

- ° You will have your own ideas about what you want to achieve. For example, you may judge your explanation of events a successful response to a client's complaint. However, it may disappoint the client if his or her expectation was that the letter would also include an outline of intended actions to prevent future occurrences.

Finally, decide on the logical sequence for presenting the information. Arrange the data in the appropriate order using bullet points. This will form the basic plan for your letter.

## 3. Drafting your letter

Write your letter for your reader:

- ° Choose your words with care. Avoid unnecessary technical terms or abbreviations, especially when writing to clients.

- Keep your sentences and vocabulary simple and straightforward.
- Be specific. For example, rather than using 'as soon as possible', give an exact date.
- Write in a tone that suits the reader and the purpose of the letter, for example using personal pronouns in response to a complaint.
- Avoid rhetorical questions. As they only have one answer, it may look as if you are trying to lead the reader to a specific conclusion.
- Keep statements positive and direct wherever possible.

*4. Editing your draft*

Once you have written your draft, you can check the content, spelling, grammar and presentation.

Use the following checklist to help you make your edits:

- ❏ Is it accurate?
- ❏ Is it logical?
- ❏ Is the information organised coherently?
- ❏ Is it clear?
- ❏ Have you addressed all the issues?
- ❏ Does it have a natural flow?
- ❏ Does it appear too brief?
  (Check you have included all the relevant details or information to support your message.)
- ❏ Does it appear overlong?
  (Remove any irrelevant material or repetitions. Try to re-phrase to make it more concise. If it is still too long, you may need to write a report or call a meeting instead.)
- ❏ Are the spelling and grammar correct? (Remember that using a computer's spellchecker is not a foolproof method.)

Once you have finished your edit you are ready to complete your final draft. Do one final proofread. This is particularly important if someone else has typed your letter.

Remember to ensure that copies of your letter go to other relevant professionals or agencies. Keep a copy on file, particularly if it relates to a client.

Below are some examples of key content for common types of letters.

### Appointment letter – key content

- Name, address and identification details (date of birth, hospital number and so on) of the client.
- Name of the clinician who will be seeing the client. (Indicate if the client may be seen by someone other than the named professional in the letter, for example, 'Mr R Johns or a member of his team'.)
- Name of the department offering the appointment.
- Address and telephone number of the clinic that the client will be attending.
- Day, date and time of appointment.
- Any instructions about preparation for the appointment. (For example, bringing a parent-held record to a baby clinic, completing a registration form, or bringing a urine sample.)
- Directions about the location of the clinic and procedures, for example, 'Book in with reception on level 2, North Wing'.
- Instructions regarding the appointment itself such as the presence of medical students.
- Details of any relevant policies, for example on non-attendance or late arrival.
- Information on how to change the appointment.
- Name, contact address and telephone number of the letter writer.
- Position and signature of the letter writer.

### Common mistakes in appointment letters

Inaccurate or out of date client address means delayed or misdirected post and appointments may be missed.

Letters where the clinic address differs from that given on the headed paper are often confusing for the client.

### Referral letter – key content

- Name, address and identification details (date of birth, hospital number and so on) of the subject of the referral.
- Date client seen by the referrer.
- Brief details of the nature of the referrer's contact with the client.
- Reason for the referral.
- Brief description of relevant clinical details (presenting symptoms, diagnosis, relevant past medical history, results of assessments or investigations or summary of intervention).
- Information on priority.
- Information on other agencies involved with the client if appropriate.
- Other relevant details about the client, for example needs an interpreter.
- Name, contact address and telephone number of referrer.
- Position and title of referrer.
- Signature of referrer.

### Common mistakes in referral letters

Letter fails to provide sufficient details to enable the receiver to prioritise the referral.

Client contact details are incomplete or out of date so it is difficult to notify the client about appointments.

Important information relating to the client is omitted, for example the client requires an interpreter or hospital transport. This can lead to missed appointments or unsatisfactory interviews.

### Letter in reply to a complaint – key content

- Name, address and identification details of complainant.
- Reason why you are writing the response (for example service manager, head of department).
- Apology (even just to say 'I am sorry to hear that you have found our service unsatisfactory').

- ○ Results of any investigations into the complaint.
- ○ Clear statements about whether the complaint is refuted or accepted, supported by the following:
  - ○ Re-iteration of any policy or guidelines in relation to the complaint.
  - ○ Completed actions in response to the complaint.
  - ○ Intended actions in response to the complaint with a timeframe for completion.
  - ○ You may want to consider heading the letter 'Without prejudice' in cases which have the potential to become litigious.
- ○ Details on any further steps the complainant may take if still dissatisfied.
- ○ Name, contact address and telephone number of letter writer.
- ○ Position and title of letter writer.
- ○ Signature.

*Common mistakes in letters about complaints*

The letter is written defensively – the clinician attempts to demonstrate his or her expertise using jargon, technical terms and excessive clinical detail.

The letter introduces irrelevant information. For example, it is not appropriate to include information about a lack of previous complaints about a health worker or a service. The complainant will only find his or her own experience of relevance.

## Reports

Clinicians regularly write clinical reports about specific clients. These are formal written accounts that are functional in nature rather than creative – the writer being required to adhere to certain recognised practices in the organisation and presentation of such material.

### Format of reports

Reports have a basic structure consisting of:

- ○ a title
- ○ an introduction

- ○ the main section
- ○ the conclusion
- ○ actions
- ○ recommendations.

*Title*

This tells the reader, at a glance, the subject matter of the report.

*Introduction*

The introduction in a report sets the scene for the reader, and makes clear the purpose of the report. It will always include specific information about where, when and why the report writer saw the client. A statement about the source of the information can also be included at this point in the report, for example observations made during direct contacts with the client, information from notes, discussion with the client's family or liaison with other professionals.

These details will help identify for the reader how and at what point the report links in with the total care for that particular client. It is also useful if the report is to be an accurate account for future reference.

In some circumstances it may be appropriate to give some background information in the introduction, for instance a brief account of the nature and length of the contact with the client. The emphasis is on brief, with the main points expressed in no more than one or two sentences. A substantial description is better placed in a separate section under a heading like 'Background Information' or 'Other Relevant Information'.

Notes about any limitations on the scope or depth of a report are also placed in the introduction (Inglis and Lewis 1982), for example if an assessment was incomplete due to the late arrival of the client.

*Main section*

Most of the information contained within a report is recorded within the main section. The content usually relates to current actions, but may refer to past or future events. It is therefore important to indicate the point in time to which the information relates, for example, 'in his previous assessment on ...'.

*Conclusion*

This is a brief paragraph that summarises the main points of the report. The conclusion to a report is often the hardest to write. It is not the place to regurgitate lines from the main body of the text, nor should it contain any new pieces of information. The writer must draw together the key messages of the report and convey these as concisely as possible. The reader will then be able to extract the key points and significant outcomes.

Actions and recommendations are usually listed at the end of the report.

*Actions*

The writer needs to make clear what actions he or she has taken or is planning to take. They are most likely to be about:

- arranging further investigations
- referral to other services
- initiating intervention
- future management of the client (for example date when client needs to be reviewed).

These need to be written in the form of specific statements that answer questions like what, why, where, when and how?

*Recommendations*

Most reports contain advice by the report writer about the management of the client. There will have been a logical development throughout the report that leads the reader to anticipate and understand this advice. Recommendations need to be presented clearly, so that they are easily identifiable to the reader. It must be clear who is expected to carry out the action and the expected timeframe. The use of a numbered list is often helpful.

*Circulation list*

One of the most useful aspects of a report is that by circulating copies, a range of different people are informed. Copies are sent to the key professionals or agencies involved with the client, for instance the client's GP would always receive a copy.

*Writing a report*

You may be about to write your first clinical report, either during your clinical practice or as part of an assignment for college. The following section offers some guidance on the four stages in constructing such a report. They are:

1.   Preparation

2.   Planning

3.   Drafting

4.   Editing.

*1. Preparation*

### Terms of reference

You may find that the timing, structure and scope of your report are to a certain extent dictated by organisational guidelines. In some circumstances there may be external factors influencing how you construct your report. For instance, an expert witness report may have to follow a set format dictated by the instructing solicitors.

Whatever the circumstances, you will still need to make certain decisions before you start preparing your report. These will include deciding on the:

- purpose of the report
- type of report
- scope of the report
- sources for gathering information for the report
- timeframe
- circulation list.

*2. Planning*

When planning your report you need to consider both its purpose and the needs of its intended readers. This will help in selecting the most relevant information and will determine the style and approach of the document.

### *What is the purpose of your report?*

Think about why you are writing the report. The most common reasons for writing a report are:

- to inform (presenting facts and figures)
- to influence (providing evidence that will persuade another person to take a specific course of action)
- to advise (offering recommendations)
- to explain (presenting interpretations)
- to record (documenting a contact)
- to summarise (providing a synopsis of the main points).

### *What information does the reader require?*

The first step in preparing a report, just like any other piece of writing, is to consider the reader. What is his or her existing knowledge and experience? This will determine how much detail you need to include and how you express your message. A comprehensive and relevant report will provide the reader with information that is both specific and in sufficient detail to meet their needs.

Avoid giving too much detail, as it will be difficult for the reader to identify the key messages. It is also likely that the report will not be read thoroughly. However, too brief a report may mean the reader will need to seek further information or, even worse, make a poor decision based on an inadequate account of the facts.

### *Organisation*

All reports, regardless of their length, need some sort of structure. The section above on the format of reports provides you with a basic framework. This will help you select and organise information into a cohesive account.

You will need to decide on appropriate headings for subdividing the content of the main body of your report. Breaking text into smaller sections in this way assists the reader in assimilating large amounts of data. The reader is also able to use headings to quickly locate specific details.

Another important consideration is the sequence in which you want information to appear in a report. Without a logical order the reader would be left struggling to work out the links between facts and figures.

There are various ways of ordering material, including:

- a temporal or chronological sequence (so past history would come before the current examination and future actions would come last)

- a developmental sequence (so information about early play would come before the development of spoken language)

- a clinical sequence (so diagnosis would come before information on intervention)

- background information to specific information (so sections about general information like education and living accommodation would come before the more specific details of an assessment).

### Gather your facts

In the same way as you would prepare a letter, you need to gather all the relevant facts and figures for your report. This information may come from the results of investigations, progress notes in the personal health record or explanations from the client. Thoroughness in record keeping will ensure that the information you use is accurate, up to date and factual. These are all requirements under the Data Protection Act (1998).

A brainstorming technique is often useful if you are dealing with a large amount of information or if you need to address a difficult subject. Write the central idea, theme or issue in the middle of a large sheet of paper. Note down ideas, opinions, facts and figures associated with the central idea using one- or two-word phrases. Join these to your keyword using lines.

The effect is to create a visual spider's web. Further details can be noted around the 'legs' of the 'spider'. Use lines and arrows to show how points link together, and to indicate the hierarchy of the information.

Once you have covered all the areas, you can start to sort your data into cohesive groupings. List key points under the relevant headings from your report. Asking yourself questions is a useful way of focusing your thinking, for example, 'How do I know this child is showing a delay in gross motor skills?' This will help you select information that will help the reader to come to the same conclusion – for example, that the child has delayed motor skills.

*3. Drafting your report*

Once you have gathered your information and organised it into a basic framework, you can start to prepare a draft. Writing a report is not just about what you say but also how you say it.

Remember that the majority of reports will now be read by the client and the client's family or carers (NHS Plan 2001). Try to phrase your report in a way that is more accessible for a lay person with limited clinical or technical knowledge. This is not to say that all terminology is to be excluded. One idea to get around this problem is to provide a summary written specifically for the client (NHS Training Division 1994).

Remember that the way in which the message is expressed often inadvertently conveys underlying attitudes. Look at this example: 'Mother initially *denied* any concerns about his hearing, but then *confessed* that she thought he did have problems…' These words imply some sort of negative judgement on the part of the report writer about the client. Check that your report is objective and your interpretations have a clear evidence base.

When preparing your final draft, consider how you will present the report. Here are some general guidelines:

- ○ Place the name or logo of the employing organisation at the top of the report.

- ○ Write a succinct title.

- ○ Place the contact address and telephone number of the report writer in the top right-hand corner.

- ○ Mark all reports containing information about clients as confidential. (Remember to mark this on the envelope as well.)

- ○ Place the client's name, address, date of birth and other identification information like a hospital or social security number in the top left-hand corner.

- ○ Date all reports. Indicate if there has been a delay between a report being dictated or drafted, and the date when it was actually typed. For instance:
  - ○ Date dictated: 21/2/01
  - ○ Date typed: 12/3/01.

○ Always sign reports. Type or print your full name, title and profession underneath your signature.

○ Number all pages. Do not repeat any headings or addresses used on the first page, but you might want to include some client identification information.

*4. Editing your report*

Once you have written your draft, you can check the content, spelling, grammar and presentation. Use the following checklist to help you make your edits.

Is the information organised? Check you have used:

❑ A clear framework

❑ A logical sequence

❑ Headings.

Is the information valid? Check the content is:

❑ Balanced (no one area is given too much emphasis)

❑ Accurate

❑ Current

❑ Objective.

Is your message clearly stated? Check that you have:

❑ Reduced unnecessary repetition

❑ Included all the key points

❑ Summarised the main points in a conclusion

❑ Clearly stated recommendations and actions.

Is the report well presented? Check:

❑ Spelling and grammar

❑ Format complies with guidelines.

Is the style appropriate? Check you have:

❑ Reduced jargon

❑ Reduced complexity

❑ Made it easy for the reader to find information

❑ Used non-judgemental language.

Once you have finished your edit you are ready to complete your final draft. Do one final proofread. This is particularly important if someone else has typed your report.

Remember to ensure that copies of your report go to other relevant professionals or agencies. Keep a copy on file in the client's personal health record.

Below are some examples of key content for common types of reports.

### Initial assessment report – key content

- ○ Name, address and identification details (date of birth, hospital number and so on) of the subject of the report.

- ○ Date client referred.

- ○ Reason for the referral.

- ○ Name and position of referrer.

- ○ Date and place where client was seen.

- ○ Details of who was present at the interview.

- ○ Details of relevant information from case history.

- ○ Name or type of assessments, tests or procedures carried out.

- ○ Results and interpretation of those assessments.

- ○ Diagnosis.

- ○ Recommendations.

- ○ Actions.

- ○ Name, title, profession and status of report writer.

### Discharge report – key content

- ○ Name, address and identification details (date of birth, hospital number and so on) of the subject of the report.

- ○ Summary of the episode of care to include:

  - ○ initial diagnosis (this allows a comparison between the client's status at admission and discharge)

  - ○ treatment provided

- outcomes (include achieved outcomes and unresolved problems)
- name of key persons involved in treatment if different from report writer.
  - Reason for discharge.
  - Date of discharge.
  - Information or instructions given to client regarding medication, therapy regimes or self-administered health care.
  - Details of circumstances that would initiate a re-referral.
  - Route for re-referral.
  - Name, title, profession and status of report writer.

**Action Points**

1. Work with a peer to examine different reports and letters. Discuss the good points. Highlight any unsatisfactory aspects. What would you change? Why? How would you change it? Now try to rewrite it using your suggestions.

---

## Summary Points

- Letters and reports about the care and management of clients are an essential form of communication within the health service.
- They are a means of conveying information, making requests, influencing decision making and confirming actions.
- Letters and reports are set out according to a standard format and often have prescribed terms of reference.

- There are four stages in writing such documents – preparation, planning, drafting and editing.

- Good writing skills involve the ability to select relevant information and organise it in a logical sequence.

- Copies of reports between health professionals are likely to be seen by the client. Careful consideration needs to be given to the choice of vocabulary and the way the message is phrased.

# 6

# Information Leaflets for Clients

There is an increasing demand from clients for information regarding their illness, care and treatment. Providing written material is one way of helping to meet this need and involving clients in decision making. However, both professionals and clients have expressed concern about the quality of some of this information. The following chapter looks at how the writing and presentation of written leaflets may be improved.

**Getting started**

Most written material benefits from a team approach to its development, writing and production. Decide at an early stage who will be part of this team. Useful members might include:

- o clinicians with relevant experience
- o researchers or academics with knowledge of current research relevant to the subject matter
- o persons with writing experience
- o representative(s) from the users (clients, clinicians, administrative staff)
- o persons with design experience.

Your team will need to:

- o establish the aims or objectives of the leaflet
- o identify the target audience
- o decide on the content, format and presentation of the material
- o choose the manner of production and distribution

- ○ determine how and when the material will be evaluated
- ○ cost the development, production, distribution and evaluation.

**Planning the content of your leaflet**

Your choice of content will be determined by your objectives, your target audience and your evidence base.

*What are your objectives?*

What do you hope your material will achieve? The purpose of written material is usually one of the following:

- ○ to increase awareness
- ○ to motivate
- ○ to change attitudes
- ○ to change behaviour
- ○ to teach a new behaviour
- ○ to teach a new skill
- ○ to offer support and advice
- ○ to give information.

Your aims will affect the type of information you choose and the way in which you present it.

*Who is your target audience?*

You need to define your target audience so that you can make the information in your leaflet relevant and useful to them. They may share an illness or other condition, or they may be linked in some other way, for example attending the same GP practice. What are their characteristics? Find out about age, gender, ethnic group, and any special needs like low literacy skills or a sensory impairment.

Once you are clear about your audience, you can start to identify their information needs. Find out the type of information they want and when they want it. For example, at what point in the care process or stage of their illness would that type of information be useful? It would also be invaluable to have their views on other written material they have used.

There are various ways of canvassing the views of clients (along with family and carers). These include using:

- questionnaires
- interviews
- focus groups[1]
- representatives from voluntary organisations or self-help groups
- representatives of local ethnic minorities.

### Establish your evidence base
Look for evidence on:

- need
- best practice
- current theory.

### Research other publications

Find out about written leaflets that have already been produced for your client group. You may find that there is perfectly adequate information already published but not accessible to your clients. For instance, a lot of very good work is produced at a local level or by other associated agencies like social services. It may be more cost-effective to buy in this material than trying to re-invent the wheel yourself.

Alternatively you may want to adapt ideas from other leaflets for the needs of your specific client group. For example, an interactive diary format used by one client group might be modified for another. Even reading leaflets where you feel the information is inadequate, incorrect or poorly presented is of use to you in your planning. You can certainly learn from other people's mistakes.

### Consult the users

Users are not just the clients but also the clinicians and administrative staff who would be using the material. Find out their views and suggestions.

---

1   Focus groups are a useful way of seeking the views of a large number of clients. A facilitator using a set agenda of topics and questions runs groups of up to ten people. The group discussion is audiotaped and analysed later.

*Consult within your organisation*

Ask the information officer in your organisation about the types of requests for information he or she receives from the public. Clinical audits might also yield some information about complaints or plaudits regarding the giving of information.

*Consult with co-agencies*

Talk with associated agencies about the materials they produce and their perspective on the topic you wish to write about.

*Look at guidelines on best practice*

Check clinical guidelines, quality standards and care pathways.

*Review the research*

Search databases and liaise with medical schools or universities for information on current research findings.

*Seek an expert opinion*

Find out from the experts about what should be in your leaflet. Use the Delphi technique. This involves a panel of experts who are asked to make suggestions about the ideal content. However, rather than discussing it as a group, the experts are asked to comment anonymously. The information is compiled into a list by a person external to the panel, who marks any items that have not received unanimous support. The list is returned to the experts who are asked to comment (again anonymously) on the items not agreed. They must give reasons why they should be included or excluded. The process is repeated until there is a core list of items that everyone agrees upon.

### Use a storyboard

A storyboard is a way of planning the sequence of your information. Using a simple grid, the planned content is plotted out like a story using simple bullet points or summaries. This gives you a clearer idea of the order and provides an overview that is difficult to get in any other way.

Try different approaches. Your instinct may be to follow the medical model and start with a description of the disease, causes, treatment and so on. However, this might not be the way in which the client experiences his or her illness. You need to start with what is most important to the client.

For instance, this might be his or her symptoms. The storyboard helps you try out different arrangements. Again, user consultation will help in planning the most appropriate sequence.

## Delivering the message

Your aim is to write a leaflet that clearly expresses its message to the intended audience. In practice, achieving readability and comprehensibility is a more difficult task than it first appears. You will need to plan carefully how you deliver your message. The important points to consider are:

- choosing vocabulary
- phrasing the message
- increasing comprehension of the message
- engaging the reader
- improving recall of information.

### *Choosing vocabulary*

As health professionals we are so familiar with medical and health jargon that we often become oblivious to its usage in our own language. It will certainly be the case that our experience of the care process will be different from that of a significant proportion of our client group. This means we need to make a conscious choice about the vocabulary we use in materials prepared for clients.

#### *Use the more common forms of expression*

Using high frequency words increases the readability of your material. For example, the words listed below on the right are more widely known and are therefore more likely to be familiar to the reader.

| | |
|---|---|
| haemorrhage | bleed |
| pharmacist | chemist |
| halitosis | bad breath |
| minimally invasive surgery | keyhole surgery |
| embolism | blood clot |
| commencement | start |

*Be consistent*

Choose one term and use this consistently throughout the leaflet, for example selecting 'bowel' to refer to the intestines and not interchanging it with other synonyms like intestines, colon or gut.

*Explain terminology*

It may be necessary to use certain terms and expressions. Always make sure you give an explanation, and if necessary provide examples. In the following extract, the term 'urethra' is explained in simple language.

> What is the prostate?
>
> The prostate is a small gland, which lies at the neck of the bladder in men and surrounds the urethra – the tube that carries urine from the bladder to the penis ...'
>
> (World Cancer Research Fund 2000)

Once you have explained a label, continue to use it rather than introducing any alternatives.

*Be aware of ambiguous word meanings*

In English some of the words we use alter in meaning depending on the context in which they are used. Clients may understand a word in one context but not in another.

Look at the examples below:

- ○ Registrar =
    - ○ In the registry office – a keeper of names for births, deaths and marriages.
    - ○ In the hospital – a senior doctor.
- ○ Raw =
    - ○ In a recipe – uncooked.
    - ○ In a test result – raw score means the sum of correct items.

Make sure that your reader will understand the intended meaning of your vocabulary.

*Check the emotional loading of words*

Certain words will have a higher emotional loading for clients. For example, the words 'cancer' and 'treatment' in a recall letter after breast screening were found to make women worry (Austoker and Ong 1994). Rewording the message may reduce stress and anxiety – so using 'most recalled women are found to have normal breasts' was more reassuring than 'most recalled women are found not to have cancer' (Ong, Austoker and Brouwer 1996). The word cancer is also avoided.

*Write words in full*

Avoid using abbreviations or acronyms even if these are explained in your text. They tend to confuse readers who are less familiar with these types of expressions.

### Phrasing the message

The type and length of sentences will affect the amount of information the reader understands and remembers.

*Use short words and sentences*

There are a number of published tests designed to calculate the readability of set pieces of text (Flesch 1948; Gunning 1952). These make their calculations using various formulae that involve looking at the length of sentences and the number of syllables. These tests predict the reading age required to cope with decoding the text. They are of use in checking the readability of your text but are not fail-safe ways of establishing how easy your text is to read. Use short words and sentences as this helps understanding and recall of information in written information (Ley 1982). Aim for a maximum of 20 words in a sentence.

*Write sentences in the active rather than the passive voice*

Active sentences are more direct and give impact to a message. Compare the following sentences:

> 'Tooth decay is prevented by regularly brushing the teeth' (passive).
>
> 'Regular brushing prevents tooth decay' (active).
>
> 'The bandage needs to be removed after two days' (passive).
>
> 'Remove the bandage after two days' (active).

*Avoid using abstract concepts*

Choose concrete terms to describe or explain abstract concepts.
   Compare the following:

| Empowerment | give choices, take control, make decisions |
| Episodes of care | your stay in hospital, the period of your therapy |
| Partnership | working together. |

*Be specific*

Make your statements specific. The use of vocabulary that requires the reader to make some sort of judgement is best avoided. For example, in the sentence, 'Make sure you have an adequate fluid intake', the reader is expected to estimate the value of 'adequate'. How do you measure adequate? The sentence might be better phrased as 'drink six glasses of water a day'. Other examples are 'excessive bleeding', 'severe pain', 'small discharge' or 'enlarged gland'. Rephrase the statements so they give the reader information about how to measure these things.

*Be succinct*

Remove any words that are superfluous to the meaning of the sentence. Are there any repetitions of words with a similar meaning? Is there a more concise way of saying your message? For instance 'one pill *every day of the week*' might be rephrased as 'a pill *daily*'.

*Be positive*

Use statements that give a positive message. For example, 'nine out of ten people make a complete recovery' is better than 'one in ten people die'.

### Increasing comprehension of the message
The way in which you phrase your message will affect how easy it is for the reader to understand the information.

*Use simple sentence constructions*

Simple sentences have more content words like nouns, verbs and adjectives that give the reader specific information. Avoid using complex sentences containing lots of small grammatical words that are not strictly necessary to the meaning. For example, 'You should eat up to about five portions of fruit and vegetables in a day' is easily converted into the simple and well-known phrase, 'Eat five portions of fruit and vegetables a day'.

### State the context first

In the following sentence the key message is about low fat foods:

> 'Vegetables and fruit are low fat foods.'

The reader is not aware of the significance of the list of foods until he reaches the end of the sentence. Place 'low fat foods' at the beginning, and the reader has a meaningful context in which to place the following list of foods.

> 'Low fat foods include vegetables and fruit.'

### Use the client's own knowledge

New information is more easily assimilated when it can be incorporated into what the client already knows. For example, give the client a list of low fat foods and ask them to circle the ones they already eat. Next, ask them to write out the names of the foods that they were unaware were low in fat. Ask them to choose, from this list, foods they would like to start eating. Get them to divide the list into completely new items and ones that could be used to replace a high fat food they currently consume. By helping the client to recognise familiar foods and highlighting new ones, you are helping them assimilate the information into their knowledge base.

### Engaging the reader

Like any piece of written work, your leaflets need to attract and maintain the reader's interest. You need to phrase your message in a way that is appealing and meaningful for the reader.

### Avoid making assumptions

Some written material may unintentionally offend when the writer has made assumptions about the reader, for instance assuming that families are two parent, or that married women stay at home or work part-time. Check that your material is free of bias.

*Address the whole person*

The language you use in your material can help to show that you see the reader as a whole person – somebody who has feelings, experiences and a life other than their condition. Avoid terms that label the person, for example, diabetic, stroke patient or depressive.

*Make your message personal*

Health information that is tailored to the specific needs, interests and concerns of individuals has been found to be more effective than generic material (Krenter *et al.* 1999). The use of pronouns like 'he', 'she' and 'you' and words that indicate male and female make the message more personal. Computers also make it much easier for the clinician to adapt materials for the individual needs of the client.

*Communicate an 'I can do this' message*

Clients are more likely to make behaviour changes when they feel they will succeed. Design your material so that the client is taken through a number of small but achievable steps.

*Use vocabulary acceptable to the client*

The way in which language is used to describe and denote groups of people carries important messages about beliefs and attitudes. Consultation with users will help you make the right choice of vocabulary and avoid offending your reader. For example, for many deaf people the term 'deaf and dumb' is not acceptable.

### Improving recall of information

The way in which you organise and present information will help the reader in remembering the key messages.

*Use short words and sentences*

Use short words and sentences as this decreases the memory load for the reader.

*Make it interactive*

Material where the client is invited to actively engage with the material is more likely to be remembered. Asking the client to do, say, write or draw are all ways of increasing his or her involvement.

Examples might be:

- Ticking a checklist –

Reasons for giving up smoking

  ❑ I want to save money

  ❑ I want to feel healthier.

- Filling in personal details on a pre-written action plan –

  Get support for your weight loss.
  Tell family and friends you are going to lose weight. Ask them for their support.
  I am going to ask _____ to help me.

- Writing a goal and choosing the date it will be achieved.

- Completing a daily diary sheet on symptoms.

- Phrasing information as questions: in answering the questions the client has more information to help them decide on a course of action.

  Client concerned about prostrate cancer –
  Do you need to pee frequently?
  Is it painful?
  Is there blood in the urine?

- Asking the client to explain a term, procedure or instruction to a friend or family member.

'Drawing' is a simple way of getting the client doing something. Nothing elaborate is required. For example:

- Drawing a circle round the names of low fat foods when presented with a list of several different types of food.

- Drawing a sad, happy or neutral face in response to a questionnaire. This could be completed pre- and post-treatment.

- Marking weight loss on a graph.

- Drawing in the hands on a series of clocks to indicate the different times to take medicines.

*Present information in chunks*

Group bits of information together that have some sort of common link – so advice on keeping warm for old people might be divided into the following groups: food and drinks, clothing, heating rooms and night-time – rather than listing a number of individual pieces of advice.

## Producing your written information

The Audit Commission (1993) found that the poor quality of some information leaflets made them impossible to read. User consultation has also criticised the lack of professionalism in the production of such materials (Duman and Farrell 2000).

The following section highlights the important factors to consider when producing printed leaflets. This will help you to recognise excellence in printed material and to describe your requirements to printers.

### *Typography*

An important consideration when you are designing written materials for clients is how you present your text on the printed page. You will need to think about the size and type of print, as well as how the text is arranged on the page. This is partly about making the written material appear interesting to the reader so that he or she will want to read it. It is also about helping to organise and present text in a way that increases its readability and makes it easier to understand.

Try the following design tips.

### *Font size*

Choose a font size of at least point size 12. Small text looks difficult to read and is an effort for some people to see.

### *Font type*

Choose a simple style of lettering. Avoid using italic or script font styles as these are more difficult to read.

### *Page Layout*

#### **Spacing**

The spaces on the printed page are as important a consideration as the text. Spaces occur either vertically (for example the spaces between headings, paragraphs and lines) or horizontally (for example the spaces around text or in the margins).

The way in which space is used on a page is one of the key factors in increasing the reader's comprehension and retrieval of information (Hartley 1980). Large blocks of closely printed text can discourage readers, especially those with literacy problems. It is also more difficult for the reader to identify key information and understand how the material is organised.

Aim to:

- o Reduce the amount of text on a page so that there is a good ratio of space to print.

- o Break up long paragraphs into short blocks of text.

- o Align text with the left-hand margin so that all lines start in a regular way.

- o Avoid justifying text so that both the right- and left-hand margins are made regular. This justification is achieved by altering the spacing between words to produce lines of equal length. The irregular spacing between words caused by this process reduces the readability of the text.

- o Indent the first line of a new paragraph using several spaces. This has been found to improve the readability of the text.

### Format of text

*Headings*: provide a structure for your text. Headings help to organise material and draw the reader's attention to salient points.

*Capitals*: avoid printing text entirely in upper case as this can slow the reader. Capitals help to guide the reader as to where sentences start and end. This function is lost when all letters are in upper case. Capitalisation may also give unintended prominence to a word or phrase (Albert and Chadwick 1992).

*Add emphasis*: use different font styles like bold or underlining to highlight key words or phrases. Enlarging text is another useful way to attract the reader's attention to important information.

*Lists*: use bullet points or numbering for listing facts, but remember that Arabic numerals like 1, 2, 3, are easier to read than Roman i, ii, iii.

*Use of illustrations*

There are a number of reasons why you might consider using illustrations:

- o   Illustrations attract attention.
  Placing a picture or photograph on the front cover of a leaflet is one way to get it noticed.

- o   Illustrations are an additional medium for getting your message across.
  The information contained in one simple visual may take a page of text to explain. They can also show details that would be difficult for a client to visualise from just a written or spoken explanation.

- o   Visual images help people remember more of the message.
  We know that people remember only about 10 per cent of what they read and 20 per cent of what they hear. People are likely to remember 30 per cent from visual images.

- o   Visual images add interest.
  Text is more appealing if combined with illustrations.

Examples of the use of illustrations include:

- o   depicting the stages in a medical procedure

- o   showing views of internal organs

- o   portraying the manifestation of a disease or infection

- o   contrasting the correct with the incorrect, for example good posture and poor posture

- o   photographs of equipment

- o   diagrams of physical exercises

- o   pictures of food groups.

Choose your illustrations with care. Ley (1988) warns that pictures may be distracting and increase anxiety. Visual images may have a high emotional impact for the client. For example, feedback from some clients about a leaflet on early detection of oral cancer indicated that pictures of oral lesions might be disturbing (Woodward and Charlton 1995).

Remember:

- o Make sure illustrations are relevant to the meaning of the text. For example, the picture on the front of a leaflet must convey a message about the content.

- o Match the format of your illustrations to your intended readers. For example, a magazine-style picture story may be more appropriate for subject matter aimed at teenagers.

- o Simple illustrations are always better. Photographs are often complex and abstract images may confuse or be misinterpreted.

- o Seek professional support when developing visual materials. Amateur attempts are nearly always below the standard required for publication. Check whether your organisation already employs a professional photographer or graphic artist. Otherwise you may have to consider the cost of an outside expert.

### Use of colour

Colour can make your material more attractive and interesting for the reader. More importantly it can help the reader to understand information faster by providing a structure and guiding his or her attention.

### Choosing colours

You need to have an understanding of the basic rules of how to use colour before you can think about using it in your material. These rules can be illustrated by the colour wheel, an idea originally developed by Isaac Newton. The wheel is based on the three pure colours of red, blue and yellow, known as the primary colours. The rest of the wheel is made up of secondary and tertiary colours. Mixing equal amounts of two primaries makes a secondary colour. For example, red and yellow make orange. Tertiary colours are made up of equal amounts of primary and secondary colours. For example, yellow added to green makes lime green. There are twelve colours in total. All other colours are derived from either mixing together the basic colours of the wheel, or adding black or white to them.

Use the following information to help guide you when choosing colours for your visuals:

- o Dark colours (black, dark blue) and warm colours (red, orange) advance or stand out. Use these to highlight or add emphasis to text or visuals.

- o Cool colours (pale blue or green) recede or fade into the background. Use these as a background colour where the text is in a dark or warm colour.

- o Colours opposite each other on the colour wheel contrast most strongly (for example red with green and yellow with blue). Use this combination to make a contrast between print and paper, for example dark blue letters on a yellow background.

Use colour to:

- o highlight key words or phrases

- o indicate headings and subheadings by using a different colour for these from the main text

- o emphasise specific information; for example, use a bright or warm colour for tips or hints

- o direct attention to the salient parts of an illustration; for example, use primary colours for key organs in a diagram of the body

- o differentiate between different parts of an illustration; for example, use different colours to differentiate between items in different food groups

- o structure information by colour coding different topics; for example text about preparing to stop smoking in a different colour from text relating to actually stopping smoking

- o show the links between headings and key points related to that heading by using the same colour for both.

Remember:

- o Aim for a strong contrast between the colour of the print and the colour of the paper. Some colour combinations make it difficult to read print, for instance yellow print on a white background.

- Avoid camouflaging effects, for example using two colours of the same tone like maroon on a pink background.

- Red and green together is unsuitable for colour-blind people.

- Use well-known colour associations where appropriate; for example, a red ribbon is associated with AIDS.

- Aim for a maximum of four colours on a page.

- Be consistent. If you have used one colour for medication then avoid using it for other text unless it also relates to drugs.

*Design tips*

- Always position illustrations alongside the relevant text.

- Avoid placing an illustration so that it cuts through a block of text. Although this is a popular design, it means the reader has more difficulty in following the line of text.

- Use colour, bold, larger print, arrows, underlining, boxes or circles to direct the reader's eye to the salient points in an illustration.

- Use captions to help the reader make sense of the illustration. Tell the reader what to look at in the picture, rather than just naming it.

## Preparing written materials for special client groups

Clients with literacy difficulties, English as a second language or a sensory impairment or may have a problem in understanding and making use of materials written in English. Therefore the needs of these clients must be considered carefully when planning such resources.

### Literacy difficulties

Ten per cent of adults in the general population have problems with reading and writing (ALBSU 1992). You may find that the percentage is even higher in your target audience.

Clients with literacy problems are likely to have the following difficulties with text.

*Engaging with the material*

Large areas of text will be off-putting and may suggest to the client that the written message is difficult to read.

*Speed in decoding the message*

When we are reading a sentence we tend to scan groups of words and decode these as a whole. In contrast, the less able reader has to read sentences word by word – a slow and tedious process. You can try this for yourself by writing a sentence on a transparent piece of paper. Get a friend to do the same and swap messages. Try to read the sentence through the back of the paper. You will probably be using the word-by-word method, which takes time and effort. How much text would you want to read like this? Probably not very much. Clients who read in this way are more likely to focus on small details and miss the overall message. It also means that longer sentences are harder to decode accurately as information at the beginning is often forgotten by the reader.

*Scanning text to select information*

The ability to skim through sections of text to find key facts and figures requires a good level of reading. For a client with basic reading skills, extracting essential information is going to be difficult if the text is lengthy and elaborate.

*Understanding different writing styles*

Writing is used for many different purposes and this is often reflected in the format and style of the piece. However, the purpose of a text is not always clear from its format, for example a list of items may be used in a variety of ways. The most common in everyday life is a shopping list, where you buy everything on the list. However, lists of words are not always used to instruct the reader to *do everything*. They are used in various ways, for example:

   o   a list of low fat foods that offer the dieter a *choice*

   o   a list of symptoms that *may or may not happen*

   o   a list of things to *avoid* when sunbathing.

The client may have limited experience of the different types of writing, and this may affect the way information is interpreted. The most common usage is likely to be the one known by the client.

*Written form versus the spoken form of English*

The sentence structure and choice of vocabulary tends to differ in the written form of English. A more formal approach is used, as opposed to the conversational style of speech. A person who reads infrequently will be less familiar with the written form, and therefore less comfortable with it.

*Abstract vocabulary*

Clients with low levels of literacy are more likely to be familiar with common terms. Less well known words tend to be more abstract and harder to interpret. The client may not know some of these terms or may have a very literal meaning for the word. For example, a client was found to understand the word chicken but not the category name 'poultry' (Doak, Doak and Root 1996).

*Visual displays of numerical information*

Clients may have difficulty with interpreting graphic displays of numerical information. Tables and graphs require the reader to make comparisons between data and recognise any patterns. The meaning is often not apparent and needs to be inferred by the reader. There is also an assumption that the reader has a basic knowledge of the underlying rules of these types of display, for instance that the 'x' axis is compared with the 'y' axis.

Here are some tips on preparing materials for clients with low literacy skills.

*Engage the reader*

- o Make the leaflet look easy to read by decreasing the amount of text and increasing the amount of space.
- o Break down information into short chunks, each containing one key message.
- o Use simple and clear illustrations that make the leaflet look more attractive and also help to explain the text.
- o Use a conversational voice rather than the more formal style of written English. Combine this with the use of personal pronouns to make the message feel more personal.

*Limit the amount of information*

- ○ Think very carefully about what you want to achieve with the leaflet. Select a few key messages rather than overloading the reader with lots of information and small details.

*Simplify your language*

- ○ Use shorter words and sentences. (Shorter words are often the more common forms of expression.)
- ○ Give examples to explain difficult vocabulary.
- ○ Use descriptions that help the reader to conjure up a mental picture of what you are trying to explain. For example, 'the uterus is the size of a small pear'.
- ○ Be specific about what behaviour you want the client to adopt rather than emphasising the facts. For example, rather than giving lots of detail about how exercise helps prevent heart disease, give specific ideas on appropriate physical activities.
- ○ Avoid the use of category words.

*Help organise information*

- ○ Use headings to break text down into more manageable chunks for the reader.
- ○ Use descriptive headings that give information about the desired behaviour, for example, 'how to keep warm'.
- ○ Use colour, enlargement and changes in font to highlight key words and phrases.
- ○ Place the most important piece of information first in a paragraph or in a sentence.

### English as a second language

The translation of written leaflets for clients into various languages is now fairly common. However, simply translating a text does not necessarily address all the issues you need to consider for clients with a different cultural and ethnic background. Cultural differences in diet, religion, health beliefs and so on need to be considered right at the start of your planning. User involvement in the development of materials is essential.

You will need to consider the following.

### Who is your target audience?

The person who makes decisions about the health care of the client may not necessarily be the client himself/herself. In some cultures it is the parents (even when children have become adults) or the male head of the family who will be making the decisions. You will need to plan your approach, language and style to engage these decision makers.

### Is the content applicable to the client group?

People from different cultural backgrounds will vary in basic everyday lifestyle issues, like diet, clothes, religion and contraception, as well as in attitudes about social issues, such as family structure, sickness and death.

### What is their experience of health care?

The client's experience of health care may be very different from the one in which you are working. For example, a school for children with special needs may have a very different connotation for the client, or he or she may come from a health care system where the idea of a prescription is unknown.

### What are their attitudes and beliefs about health care?

Clients may hold a certain view about how a health professional should behave and the role of the client in getting better. For example, do they see the health professional as the person making all the decisions?

### What learning styles are common in the culture?

Approaches to learning vary between cultures and this may influence how material is presented. For instance, drawings may be held in high regard in one culture whereas another may view their use in materials as childish and degrading.

### Is the translation accurate?

We can all quote examples we have seen or heard of comic errors in translation. However, such errors in translation of health material may be more serious in their effect. A back translation, although costly, is probably the best way of ensuring that details are correct and that there are no omissions in the material.

*Can the material be translated?*

Another less common problem is that some languages do not have a written form.

### Sensory impairment

Written material is a potential problem for clients with a visual impairment. Use large print and bright colours that contrast strongly with each other to help make text and visuals legible. Advice can be sought from the Royal National Institute for the Blind on how to prepare materials. Alternatives might be to have material translated into Braille or to use an audio recording. However, the cost of these methods would have to be considered carefully in relation to the need.

## Evaluation

It is crucial to incorporate a system of evaluation into your project. This will help improve the planning and execution of your present task as well as providing valuable insight for use in any future projects.

There are three main areas that require appraisal:

1.   The development stage

2.   The validity of your written material

3.   The effectiveness of your written material.

### 1. The development stage

A system for continuous review of the development process needs to be scheduled right at the start of your project. You will want to evaluate:

(a)   Timescales

(b)   Costs

(c)   Resources

(d)   Development team

(e)   Development process.

### (a) Timescales

Keep a record of the timescales required at each stage of development. Were these longer or shorter than expected? What factors were affecting timescales? Would you do anything differently?

*(b) Costs*

Developing written materials is a costly process. There are the obvious expenditures on materials and production. However, there are hidden costs that need to be accounted for when calculating the overall expense. For instance, a one-hour planning meeting with four people is equivalent to four hours in terms of salaries.

*(c) Resources*

Consider both the materials and the resources required to produce the materials. Continuous review of expenditure is needed if costs are not to escalate beyond your planned budget. Were all the resources that you required readily available, for example access to an evidence base via a library or a graphic artist for illustrations?

*(d) Development team*

Who is involved in your project? Is the composition of the team appropriate? Were there staff members who needed to be there but were not? Do different people need to be involved at different stages?

*(e) Development process*

Factors to consider might range from user involvement and methods for obtaining expert opinion to the decision making process of your team. The emphasis is on how you developed the materials and whether these procedures worked well.

**2. The validity of your written material**
Use the following checklist to help in evaluating the validity of your written material:

- ❏  Is it accurate?
- ❏  Is it relevant?
- ❏  Is it current?
- ❏  Is the intended message clear?
- ❏  Is the message believable?
- ❏  Is it interesting?
- ❏  Is it informative?
- ❏  Has it got a sound evidence base?

### 3. The effectiveness of your written material

Evaluate the outcomes of your project. A first review might be best 12 months after the completion of your project. Look back at your original objectives. Have they been achieved? This is a fundamental question but not necessarily one that is easy to answer. There are a number of different methods you can use to help you evaluate the effectiveness of your written material.

Try one or a combination of the following ways:

- ○ User feedback from clients, clinicians and administrative staff. Feedback might be obtained via focus groups, questionnaires or more general sources like the organisation's information officer.

- ○ Formalised research methods (for example randomised control trials).

- ○ Clinical audit (for example a reduction in complaints about a lack of information).

Such reviews need to continue and must be scheduled in advance. Putting a date for review on material is one way of helping to ensure this happens at the right time. The purpose of these reviews will be:

- ○ to update the information with current knowledge and practice

- ○ to monitor accessibility

- ○ to review the timing of the delivery of the information

- ○ to update the information to reflect changes in legislation

- ○ to update the information to reflect current health and social policies

- ○ to amend any inaccuracies.

You will need to decide who has responsibility for carrying out these reviews and make contingency plans in the event of staff changes.

## Summary Points

- Most written material benefits from a team approach to its development, writing and production.

- Team members would benefit from having the relevant clinical knowledge, research, writing or design experience.

- User involvement is essential at every stage of the process.

- Use common vocabulary or explain terminology. Be aware of possible ambiguities or words with high emotional impact.

- Use short words and simple sentences. Write in the active not the passive.

- Reflect the client's own knowledge and experience in your material.

- Engage the reader by addressing him or her in a personal manner that recognises him or her as a whole person. Avoid making assumptions or having a bias.

- Increase the recall of information by making your material interactive and grouping information together.

- Choose at least font size 12 and a simple style for lettering.

- The way space is used on the page is a key factor in increasing the reader's comprehension and retrieval of information.

- Use illustrations to attract attention and as another medium for getting your message across.

- Adapt your materials to meet the needs of special client groups.

- Incorporate a system of evaluation into your project and set a date for reviewing your leaflet.

## PART TWO

# Writing for Teaching and Learning

# Writing for Teaching and Learning

Teaching and learning is an integral part of the health professional's working life. All clinicians have to undergo formal training and assessment in order to obtain a qualification. Note-taking, writing essays and completing exams are familiar student activities. Once qualified the clinician is likely to return periodically to the learner role, either by attending continuing education programmes or, more formally, by enrolling as a postgraduate student. In addition, many clinicians are now involved as educators themselves and are writing teaching materials, and setting and marking coursework.

The main section of this part looks at writing as a learning medium and preparing materials for teaching. It includes advice on how and where to search for information and the use of effective reading strategies – skills that are of use not only to the student but also to clinicians wishing to review the literature either for research purposes or to establish an evidence base. The second section of this part gives some specific advice on using written materials in teaching.

The final section covers several writing activities from note-taking, essays and assessment through to dissertations and research.

## Writing as an Aid to Learning

Types of information. Finding information. Effective reading. Writing introductions, explanations and conclusions.

## Preparing Materials for Teaching

The purpose of teaching materials. Planning how to use materials. Making choices. Preparing and using overheads, slides, flipcharts and handouts.

# Teaching and Learning Skills in Context

### Note-taking

The purpose of note-taking. Different styles of note-taking. Note-taking in different contexts. Organisation and filing of notes.

### Essays

Purpose of essays. Analysing an essay title. Planning an outline. Writing a draft. Assessment criteria.

### Assessment

Summative assessments. Preparation. Use of mind maps. In the exam.

### Dissertations

The characteristics of a dissertation. Choosing a title. Styles of referencing.

### Research projects

Structure of quantitative and qualitative research papers. Displaying numerical data.

# 7

# Writing for Teaching and Learning
## Writing as an Aid to Learning

Writing is a dynamic process in which the written word is the end point. Writing an academic piece of work will take the following steps:

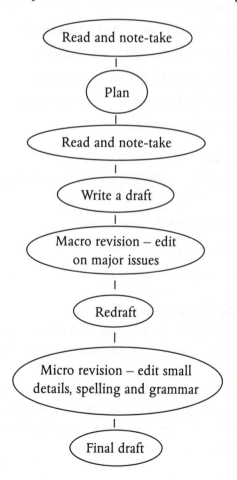

Individual writers may spend longer on certain stages and may repeat steps. For example, one person may do several drafts before they are satisfied that the work is finally ready. Another may be continually reading and adding material right up to the point of the final draft.

During the writing process you will learn how to:

○ search for data

○ appraise the quality and validity of material by other writers

○ recognise the significance of material both in general terms and for the purposes of your writing

○ select relevant information

○ collate large amounts of information

○ recognise the connections between different sets of information

○ organise thoughts into a logical and coherent account

○ construct a written argument or opinion

○ write using an academic style of writing

○ write to a deadline and within a specified word limit

○ present written material.

## Finding information

You need to develop a systematic approach to searching for information. Think about:

1.   The type of information you need

2.   Where you can find information

3.   How you search for information.

### 1. What type of information do you need?

Decide on the type of information you need for your studies. Remember material might be in printed form, on microfilm, microfiche, CD-ROM or online.

○ Definitions – look in specialist dictionaries for an explanation of terms. Further clarification of these terms can be gained by using introductory texts and review articles where the words will be used in a meaningful context.

○ An overview of the topic – use an introductory text, a review or general article in a professional journal.

○ Seminal works – look out for seminal works; these are texts recognised by the experts as essential reading. You will find that they frequently appear in the reference list of different articles and books. A literature review would certainly make a reference to them, and your tutor may also give you guidance about this.

○ Detailed coverage of the topic – look in specialist textbooks or read in-depth journal articles that focus on a particular area.

○ Original research – read research papers published in peer-reviewed journals or in conference reports. Unpublished theses and research in progress may also be useful to you:

　　○ Unpublished theses will be held in the library of the relevant academic institution. Find out about the topics of the theses by contacting the librarian or accessing the database 'Index to theses'. This is available on the Internet at *www.theses.com* and it lists all the theses accepted by UK universities.

　　○ Use the database 'Current Research in Britain' (CRIB) to find out about research in progress at academic institutions in the UK. It is available on the Internet at *crib.cos.com*, on CD-ROM or in printed form.

○ Procedures or processes – look out for information provided on video, audio cassette or multimedia. Training packages are also likely to cover 'how' you do things.

○ Medical illustrations – use illustrated anatomy books, slides and video. Check out websites like *www.medscape.com* or the National Electronic Library for Health at *www.nelh.nhs.uk* that have medical imaging.

○ Statistics – check out publications from local authorities, health authorities, government departments and relevant voluntary organisations. Look at 'National Statistics' via the website *www.statistics.gov.uk*.

- Legislation and government policies – your main source will be Her Majesty's Stationery Office. Its website is *www.legislation.hmso.gov.uk*. You can also check publications from the Department of Health via *www.doh.gov.uk/publications/index.html*.

- Clinical guidelines – find out about publications on this subject by the relevant professional body. For example, the Royal College of Speech and Language Therapists publishes *Clinical Guidelines by Consensus for Speech and Language Therapists*. A search using the keywords 'care pathways' or 'clinical pathways' along with the relevant topic will produce some useful information on this topic.

- Clinical experience, roles and responsibilities – find suitable articles in professional journals or use books designed to give practical advice on clinical issues or roles.

- Current opinion – look for articles in professional journals.

- News stories – read the newspapers held at the library or access websites like *www.reutershealth.com*.

### 2. Where can you find information?

The two main places to find information are libraries and the Internet.

### Libraries

There are various libraries that you can access.

- Your local library – find out if it has a reference section.

- A national library – the British Library, for example.

- A specialist library – some libraries specialise in certain aspects of health care. For instance, the King's Fund library at *www.kingsfund.org.uk* has material on health care management, health economics and social policies. The information service of the Wellcome Trust at *www.wellcome.ac.uk* focuses on medical history.

- Libraries run by voluntary organisations – some of these associations have an information service. For example, the Royal National Institute for Deaf People at *www.ucl.ac.uk* has a library.

- o  Electronic Libraries – check out libraries available on the Internet. For example, the Cochrane Collaboration has a library at *hiru.mcmaster.ca/cochrane/* or try the National Electronic Library for Health at *www.nelh.nhs.uk.*

- o  Libraries that are part of professional associations – are you already qualified and studying as a postgraduate student or doing a continuing education programme? Check whether your professional body has a library available to its members. For example, the Royal Society of Medicine, the Royal College of Nursing and the British Medical Association all have libraries open to their members. Non-members may apply for temporary membership on payment of a fee; however, access to the library facilities is often restricted to reference use only.

- o  Alumni – you may be able to visit your old college or university library.

- o  Links via your employer – are you continuing to work as well as study? Check whether you have access to any libraries through your employer. Most large organisations are involved in both undergraduate training and continuing education programmes. They are likely to have either on-site resources to support these courses or links with a further or higher education establishment. Libraries are often part of the postgraduate centre, nursing school or medical school.

*The Internet*

The Internet gives you the opportunity to conduct database searches, read online journals and access information via numerous health-related websites. However, you do have to be cautious when using the Internet. Always consider the credibility of the person or organisation that has set up any website you are using.

### 3. How do you search for information?

*Catalogues and indexes*

All libraries have some form of cataloguing system that lists the resources in the library. This will be either a manual system, usually in the form of a card index, or electronic, using computers with online catalogues.

The catalogue system will allow you to search by author, title or keyword. It will tell you:

- the number of copies held by the library
- the location of books (shows a classification number)
- availability (Is it on loan? Missing? Overdue?)
- type of loan (Reference? Seven day?).

Use the library catalogue to carry out basic searches. For a more comprehensive search, use one of the published indexes that lists books or journals by subject. For example, MEDLINE is a clinical medical database compiled by the National Library of Medicine in the United States of America. Most of these indexes are now available in a variety of formats (printed, online and CD-ROM). Some are also available via the Internet.

Some useful databases are MEDLINE, CINAHL – Cumulative Index to Nursing and Allied Health Literature (USA) – ClinPSYC, PsychLit and CANCERLIT.

References to the literature are held on a record divided into fields. Each of these fields will contain key information, such as the title and author of an article, as well as the year of publication, the source journal and an abstract.

Electronic searches are faster and more effective, particularly if you want to access several databases. The full text of some journals is available on the Internet; however, for access to many articles you will have to find the original journal. Libraries hold different sets of periodicals, so join ones that give you access to your preferred titles.

### Identify your search terms

You may have been given a start in your search for information in the form of a directed reading list. Books and articles will lead you to other sources via their reference lists. Articles will also give a list of key terms that will be of use to you in searching for similar material. However, you will still need to plan your search in order to be effective and achieve the best results.

Start by identifying the problem or question you would like answered. Write this out in a sentence and then select the keywords. These will be the topics, themes or concepts you will use as your search terms. It may be helpful to think of a list of synonyms to use as alternatives.

*Refine your search*

The key to a successful search is the ability to narrow the field of enquiry. Think about the type of information you require. Is it legislation? Is it research? This will affect where you look for the information. Use time periods and geographical areas to help limit the extent of your search, for example searching a database for articles published after 1990 or only those from America and the United Kingdom.

*Manage your time*

Plan your schedule. How much time do you have available to do the search? Do you have to book a terminal at the library in advance? What percentage of your overall study time have you allocated to collecting information? Prioritise your reading so that you have covered any recommended or seminal texts first. Remember there is no point in accumulating lots of photocopies of book chapters or articles if you have no time to read them.

*Searching on an electronic database*

Searching an electronic database is one of the quickest ways of finding information. Get some basic training in retrieving results before you start. This can often be arranged via the library staff, or help is sometimes offered online.

Remember these general search strategies:

- Select the terms that represent the most important concept or theme in your subject.

- Understand how your database is indexed. Some databases are indexed using a restricted thesaurus of terms; others allow a search using free text words or a combination of both. You are likely to be more successful if you use terms from the thesaurus, so check these out in advance.

- Avoid terms that are very general, as these will create too many references (often thousands!). Conversely, too narrow a term may generate only a few or even no references at all.

- Use 'explode' to find the subdivisions of your chosen term. It may be more productive to search with one of these words.

- Only use content words. Leave out function words like 'the', 'and' and 'a' as these will not be recognised as valid search terms.

- Search via different fields, for example by title or year of publication.

- Remember that some databases may use American spelling.

- Make use of synonyms, as the terms recognised by the database may be different from the ones you are inputting. For example, the database may recognise the term 'adverse effects' rather than 'side effects'.

- Check the keywords listed on the articles you have found. Is there a common set of terms you can use?

- For databases that use Boolean logic:

    - To broaden your search, use 'OR' to combine two or more terms. This will find articles and books that have one, two or more of the terms.

    - To narrow your search use 'AND' to combine two or more search terms. This will only search for articles that have all of the terms connected by 'AND'.

    - To exclude information, use 'NOT' to combine two search terms. The second term will be specifically excluded from the term.

- Keep a note of successful search strategies.

At the end of your search, save the references you have retrieved, either on disk or as a print-out.

**Effective reading**

Your search will have highlighted some useful books or articles to read. You now need to make sure that you are effective in selecting the pertinent information from these sources.

Start by taking a few minutes to get to know the material:
For books find out:

- How is the book arranged?
  Use the contents list to see how information is organised.

- How is it meant to be used?
  Look at the user's guide or in the introduction.

- What type of information does it contain?
  Practical advice, case studies, research studies or theory.

- What is it about?
  Get a general idea of the topics by skimming the headings, introductions and summaries.

- What is the level of the book?
  Introductory, advanced, for the novice or the specialist.

- Who is the author?
  Read the author description to find out about his or her background and experience.

For articles find out:

- What is it about?
  Read the abstract first to decide if it is relevant to your needs.

- What are the keywords?
  Articles should provide a list of keywords. These terms will help you in searching for similar articles.

- How long is it?
  You may need to copy longer articles. See 'How does the copyright law affect photocopying?' in Chapter 19.

- What type of references?
  What sources has the author used? How many references are there?

Make your reading purposeful by thinking of questions that you would like the text to answer. This will help you select relevant information rather than making a précis of a whole chapter or article.

Then read through a section at a time. What points is the author trying to make? Is it about concepts, principles or a general description? Take notes after you have read each section and not line by line. Keep referring back to your questions so you only select the information you need to help answer your queries.

Take time out to reflect on what you are reading and the information you have noted. How does it relate to what you know already? Does it confirm or contradict your views? What does it add to your knowledge base? What information is missing?

As well as reflecting on your reading, you also need to review your progress at regular intervals. Can you summarise the main points? This will keep you alert and on the right track.

### Critically appraising the information

It is important that you develop the skills to appraise the material you are reading.

- Is it current? Look at the date of publication but also at the date of the references. (Remember that books, due to the time it takes to produce them, are published a few months after they are written. Journals will have more up-to-date information.)

- What evidence base are the authors using? Is it based on primary sources of information like research studies? Does it refer to seminal texts in the field? What is the range of literature in the reference list?

- What is new information to you? Make a note of any material that is fresh or additional to what you know already.

- Do you agree with the authors? Does it contradict what you have read before?

- Is it accurate? Does it contain contradictions or anomalies?

- Is it unbiased? Do the authors take a particular stance on an issue? Is this stated overtly by the authors or inferred from the text?

- What use is the information? Think about how you might apply it to clinical practice.

Use the following checklist when appraising research papers:
Literature review

- ❑ Is the literature chosen for review relevant to the research question?

- ❑ How current is the material?

- ❑ Does it include references to seminal works?

- ❑ How broad is the literature review? (For example, is there a range of studies from a wide time period, different countries of origin?)
- ❑ Has the writer attempted to analyse and evaluate the literature? Or is it merely a description of various studies?

Research design

- ❑ Does the design fit the research question being asked?
- ❑ Do you agree with the rationale given for the choice of design?

Methodology

- ❑ Is the collection of data systematic and objective?
- ❑ Is there enough detail? (A good test is whether you could replicate the study using only the information in the paper.)
- ❑ Is there enough information about the subjects? (A rule of thumb is the fewer the subjects in the study, the greater the amount of information about them.)

Results

- ❑ Is the reporting objective?
- ❑ Is all the key data represented?
- ❑ What do the results tell you?
- ❑ Do you agree with the choice of statistical analysis?

Discussion

- ❑ Do the results support the author's interpretations?
- ❑ Have the authors offered an objective evaluation of their research (both strengths and weaknesses)?
- ❑ Are the findings relevant for clinical practice or theoretical knowledge? (What use could you make of the information?)

Make use of any systematic reviews you see published in journals. You can also access information about reviews via the Cochrane Collaboration at *hiru.mcmaster.ca/cochrane/* and the NHS Centre for Reviews and Dissemination (York University) via *www.york.ac.uk/inst/crd/*.

**Writing skills**

Once you have gathered all your information and organised it into a suitable structure, your next step is the actual writing. The following section looks at the 'how' of written work. Use it in conjunction with Chapter 16, 'Determining Your Style'.

*Writing an introduction*

The reader, like the listener in a conversation, needs some opening statements to introduce him or her to the forthcoming topic. The content of this introduction will vary between different types of written composition – so the introduction to an essay will differ from that of a research project.

A good introduction will arouse the interest of the reader and make him or her want to read further. It is this element of an introductory paragraph that is the most difficult to perfect. Devices such as quotes, examples, questions or controversial statements might be used to create an original and interesting start to a composition. However, these methods need to be used with caution.

In general:

- Avoid overwhelming the reader with too many themes in the introduction.

- Choose quotes or examples that are relevant to your topic.

- Remember that devices such as quotes, examples and controversial statements are not meant to stand alone.

*Writing explanations*

Explanations are used to:

- give information

- clarify

- provide reasons.

Brown (1978) identified three main types of explanation:

1. Descriptive (how?)
   This type of explanation provides a straightforward description of structures, procedures and processes. For example, how is a database set up? How is blood pressure recorded?

2.  Interpretative (what?)
    This type of explanation offers a definition of terms or seeks to clarify an issue. For example, what is the Data Protection Act (1998)? What do the results of a blood test mean?

3.  Reason giving (why?)
    This type of explanation attempts to give reasons. This often involves the discussion of principles, values and motives. For example, why do we need supervision?

Plan how you will write your explanation:

1.  Identify what you want to explain. It is useful to start by phrasing your explanation as a what, how or why question:

    o  *What* is an erythrocyte?

    o  *How* do you measure blood pressure?

    o  *Why* do people develop anaemia?

2.  What are the key elements?
    Identify the hidden variables or key points within the explanation (Brown 1978). For example, in '*What* is an erythrocyte?', the variables are the structure, (including size and shape), function, location and formation. You may want to include information on haemoglobin and blood groups.

3.  What is the relationship between these elements?
    In the above example, your explanation would include the relationship between the structure of the cell and its function and location in the body.

Once you have identified the key elements, you can start to think about how you will organise the information. This is about how you cluster and sequence the facts. Start with the most important items and work your way through to the least important. Signal to the reader which points are major and therefore more significant. Use cue phrases like 'it plays an essential role in...' or 'the fundamental point to remember...'.

It is difficult to understand the detail until we have the whole picture, so start with broad areas and gradually narrow these down to specific points (Shimoda 1994). For example, in a description of erythrocytes, you might want to start with a few sentences about blood. 'Blood transports oxygen and nutrients to the body tissues and takes away carbon dioxide and other wastes. The colourless fluid of the blood, known as plasma, carries amongst other cells erythrocytes or red blood cells. Erythrocytes are...'

### Using examples

Use examples as part of your explanations to illustrate or help to clarify a point. Students need to avoid the standard textbook ones, as tutors will be only too familiar with these. Use case studies or examples from clinical practice as these are particularly effective.

### Using quotes

Quotes are extracts reproduced from other texts. The wording must be exact and a reference provided to indicate the source.

Use quotes:

- to corroborate (for example statistical evidence)
- to give authority
- to illustrate
- to help explain
- to add new information
- to provide interest
- to make use of a unique expression.

When using a quote:

- Use the exact wording from the original. Any modifications to the wording must be placed within square brackets.
- Shorter quotations are included within the body of the text, and are enclosed by single quotation marks.
- Longer quotes are usually set apart from the main text of the page, and indented from the left margin.
- Always indicate the source along with the page number for the original piece.
- Use sparingly. Consider paraphrasing where possible.

### Paraphrasing

This is where an original text is rephrased by the writer in his or her own words. Paraphrasing is a common way of referring to material from other sources. However, in order to fully understand the original, the writer must be effective in interpreting the material. Remember you still need to acknowledge your source by providing a reference.

### Writing a summary

Written summaries are a brief and concise review of the main points extracted from a longer composition. The conclusion at the end of a piece of writing often contains a summary. They are also used within the main body of the text before a topic shift. These periodic reviews of the content help consolidate the reader's understanding and add emphasis to the writer's message.

When writing a summary:

- o   Make sure you select the key points or identify the essence of the message.
- o   Keep your language simple and straightforward.

### Writing a conclusion

The conclusion forms the final part of a piece of writing and helps bring it to a satisfactory closure.

A conclusion might contain:

- o   a summary of the main points (for example in a descriptive answer to an essay question)
- o   the general application of what has been discussed (for example the implications of a research project for clinical practice)
- o   a resolution to an argument (for example the writer proposes an answer to the questions or discussion points set within a dissertation)
- o   a link to the broader context (for example at the end of a dissertation, the writer might highlight the relevance of the issues under discussion to social policy).

When writing a conclusion:

- o   Avoid writing explanations, detailed analyses or new information in the conclusion.

- ○ Make a link in some way to your introductory paragraph. For example, 'we set out to examine the question of...'. This helps to bring the writing in a full circle.

- ○ Plan your endings. Allow time to complete your conclusion and allocate it a sufficient proportion of your total word limit.

**Action Points**

1. When you join a library spend some time reading the library guides to find out how the library is organised and about the classification system for books and other resources.

2. Reading through several texts can be tedious, so think of ways to make it more interesting. Try:

   - ○ Identifying the questions the writer set out to answer. How well has the writer answered these questions?

   - ○ Comparing the information with your clinical or general life experience. Write down information that you would like to follow up through clinical observation or other practical ways.

   - ○ Writing down counter arguments.

   - ○ Thinking about the attitudes the writer holds. Do you agree with them?

---

### Summary Points

- ○ Writing is a dynamic process in which the written word is the end point.

- ○ A writer will learn about searching for data and critical appraisal as well as how to construct a logical and coherent written account.

- ○ Libraries and the Internet are the two main sources of information.

- Your search for information needs to be systematic, using the terms that represent the most important concept or theme in your subject.

- Thinking of questions that you would like the text to answer is one way of making your reading purposeful.

- It is important that you develop the skills to appraise the material you are reading.

- Evaluate the validity and reliability of the material you read.

- A written account needs some opening statements to introduce the reader to the forthcoming topic.

- Explanations are often used to help clarify or describe a point.

- There are three main types of explanation: descriptive, interpretative and reason giving.

- Use examples and quotes as part of your explanations to illustrate or help to clarify a point.

- The conclusion forms the final part of a piece of writing and helps bring it to a satisfactory closure.

# 8

# Preparing Materials for Teaching

Most trainers or educators will need some kind of additional written material to support their teaching. This might be in the form of a written handout or text and visuals that are presented using overhead projectors, slide projectors, whiteboards or flipcharts.

Consider using these teaching materials to:

1.  Add interest

2.  Maintain attention

3.  Help recall of information

4.  Increase understanding

5.  Provide a structure.

1. Add interest to your presentation
Keep your audience interested by presenting information in different formats.

2. Maintain your students' attention
The attention and concentration of your students will not remain at the same level throughout your teaching session. Attention tends to decrease after the first ten minutes (Bligh 1983). It continues to fall until it reaches the lowest point half an hour into your lecture or seminar. Varying your presentation style by showing an overhead or using a flipchart is a useful way of gaining students' attention at these points (Gibbs 1992).

3. Help students remember information
We know that people remember only 10 per cent of what they read and 20 per cent of what they hear. They are likely to remember 30 per cent from

visual images, which is increased to 50 per cent when this is combined with listening. If you want to get your message across, *say* it and *show* it.

4. Increase understanding of your message
Written teaching materials provide an additional means of giving explanations, examples, background facts and figures.

5. Provide structure both for the students and yourself
Overheads and handouts are useful as an aide-mémoire for the presenter and form a framework to support the spoken message.

## Planning
Before deciding on the teaching materials you would like to use, you need to have done some essential decision making.

### *Know your objectives*
Be specific about what you want to have achieved by the end of your teaching session.

### *Determine the learning outcomes*
What are the learning outcomes for the students?

- Is it an increase in knowledge?

- Is it learning a new skill?

- Is it the ability to apply theory to a practical context?

- Is it to have a greater understanding (be able to analyse or to critically appraise information)?

- Is it the ability to integrate different facts and figures in order to formulate solutions?

- Is it a greater awareness?

### *Decide on the content*
What information is essential to make sure you fulfil your objectives and ensure the students' learning outcomes are achieved?

### *Draw up a session plan*
In what order will you present information? Decide on the sequence for presenting your content.

### How to deliver the message

You now have a plan for your session. The next stage is to decide *how* you want to put your message across. This is the stage at which you will start to think about the teaching materials you will use to help you deliver this message.

### Making a choice

Remember the purpose of teaching materials. They can:

- ○ Reinforce – use them to present your message using different formats.
- ○ Explain – use examples and analogies to help clarify details and illustrate the meaning of your spoken message.
- ○ Corroborate – use them to provide evidence to support your arguments.
- ○ Give impact – make your message memorable.
- ○ Alert – arouse the interest of the audience and thereby their attention to your message.
- ○ Persuade – use them to provide evidence to change students' attitudes, perception or beliefs.
- ○ Communicate effectively – use simple visuals to convey complex ideas that would take a page of text to explain.

Look through your session plan and identify where you might want to use some additional teaching material. For example, we know students' attention is low 30 minutes into a session, so material designed to alert might be of use at this point. At another point you may want to show a graph as evidence to support your spoken message.

### Think about resources

What equipment do you need? Is it available for you to use? There is no point in preparing slides if another lecturer has booked the projector or there is no way of dimming the lights in the teaching room.

### Consider timescales

Designing teaching materials is one of the most time-consuming aspects of preparing for a teaching session. Check that you have enough time to put together your materials. This is particularly important if you rely on somebody else to do your typing or your photocopying. Aim to make your materials reusable and suitable for a variety of contexts.

### Design your materials for your students

*Students with special needs* – a student with a visual impairment may need written or pictorial material adapted or an alternative provided.

*Gender differences* – there may be differences between men and women in how they assimilate information. A study by Togo and Hood in 1992 showed female students did less well than their male peers when information was presented exclusively in a graphic format. Another group of women who were given information conveyed by both text and graphics did better. These results suggest that the use of a mixture of text and visuals might be more suitable for a group of mixed gender students.

Always refer back to your original plan when making your final decisions on your choice of material.

Check:

- How will it help me achieve my teaching objectives?
- How will it help the students achieve their learning outcomes?
- Is it relevant to the content of my session?
- When will I use it during the session?

### General guidelines for using teaching materials

#### Support the spoken word

Remember that your acetate, slide or handout is there to reinforce your spoken message. It is not meant to be a written duplicate of your oral presentation. Always ask yourself – is this slide, acetate or handout absolutely necessary? It must add information, help explain a point or illustrate the message you are trying to convey through speech.

#### Pace your presentation

Use your materials at well-spaced intervals in order to increase interest and gain maximum impact.

*Vary your materials.*

You can add interest by varying the format of your materials. Experiment with presenting information in different ways.

### Use colour with effect

Colour can add interest and help the audience understand information faster. It can help structure your material and guide the audience's attention.

Use dark colours (like black, dark green or blue) and warm colours (like red or orange) that advance or stand out to:

- highlight key information
- indicate headings and subheadings
- emphasise the significance of an item
- make a small drawing or part of a larger drawing stand out.

Use cool colours (like pale blue or green) that recede:

- as a background colour
- on words or numerals that have less importance
- for large items or areas.

Remember:

- Use a maximum of four colours on a visual.
- Avoid red and green together because of colour blindness.
- Be consistent. Use the same colours for the same items throughout your visuals, for example green for population figures, drugs in red.

### Overhead projector

An overhead projector, or OHP, projects written or printed images from acetate sheets onto a screen in an enlarged form. It is the most flexible and widely used of all the audiovisual aids. Acetates are easy to prepare and are useful for displaying numerical information as well as text. These may be pre-prepared or handwritten straight onto the acetate during a teaching session.

The main consideration when using an OHP is that there is a limit to the amount of information that can be clearly portrayed at any one time. Too much text means having to use smaller print in order to fit it onto the acetate. This will be difficult to read from a distance and requires more time for students to assimilate all the details. It is therefore important when preparing acetates that you make text legible and restrict the amount of data. OHPs are best when used with an audience of between 10 and 50 students.

When preparing your acetates remember to:

- Limit text to a maximum of six to ten lines.

- Place text in a central position on the acetate (the lower edge of an acetate is often obscured).

- Make letters at least font size 24.

- Choose a simple style for lettering that has fairly broad strokes. It needs to be of medium density or in bold.

- Use a mixture of upper- and lower-case letters. Only put letters in capitals when labelling graphics or where there is a mixture of letters and numerals.

- Use a change in font style to highlight key points or to add visual interest, but restrict these to a maximum of two on each visual.

When using an overhead projector remember to:

- Check that the projected image is in focus and is visible from the back of the room. Do this before you start your session.

- Let the audience see the whole of the acetate at least once, and then use a piece of paper to mask out material until you are ready to present it. This helps to focus the audience's attention and controls the pace of the presentation.

- Highlight points or add information by writing on a clear acetate placed over your original. This technique can be used to build up a complex overhead from two or three simple ones. Alternatively you can slide your acetate under the roll of acetate on the machine and write on this.

- Devise a system for ordering your acetates. Always know where you put your last acetate, and where to get the next one. Filing acetates in a ring binder is one of the most effective ways of keeping them tidy.

- Switch off the OHP when you have finished showing your acetates. Never leave a blank screen.

### Slide projector

A slide projector, like the OHP, projects images onto a screen. Slides are the source of the image, rather than an acetate, and are particularly useful for portraying certain material, for example histology slides. They are preferable to the OHP when lecturing to an audience of 50 or more students.

When preparing your slides remember to:

- Limit text to a maximum of six to ten lines.

- Place text in a central position on the slide.

- Make letters large enough to be visible from the back of the room. You may have to make a dummy slide and try out different font sizes.

- Choose a simple style for lettering that has fairly broad strokes. It needs to be of medium density or in bold.

- Use a mixture of upper- and lower-case letters. Only put letters in capitals when labelling graphics or where there is a mixture of letters and numerals.

- Use a change in font style to highlight key points or to add visual interest. Restrict these to a maximum of two on each slide.

- Choose the colour of your slides with care.

  - Black text on a white background is easy to read and visible with fairly light conditions. However, it can cause eyestrain.

  - White text on a black background needs very dark conditions to be readable.

  - Blue text on a white background is easier on the eye, but needs a moderately dark room to be visible.

○ Blue on white is probably the best choice if you have a large number of slides to show.

○ Use different coloured backgrounds to indicate a change in topic. However, beware of camouflaging effects (maroon text on a pink background, for instance).

○ Substitute a complex slide with a sequence of two or three simpler versions.

When using a slide projector remember to:

○ Try out the equipment beforehand whenever possible as a projector is one of the more complicated pieces of audiovisual equipment.

○ Keep the projector lights off when placing or removing slides.

○ Make sure the lighting in the room can be dimmed and the windows blacked out.

○ Use a technique called 'masking down' to highlight key information. This involves lowlighting information not essential to the message, for example material already covered by the presenter.

○ If resources allow, have two sets of slides. You will then have a duplicate slide ready to slot in if a vital original goes missing.

○ Prior to your teaching session, use your session plan to check that you have all your slides and that they are filed in the correct sequence.

○ Never search backwards and forwards for a missing slide whilst the projector is on.

### Whiteboard (or dry write board)

A whiteboard has a number of uses ranging from a notepad for recording spontaneous comments to a sketchpad for drawing pictures and diagrams to illustrate a point. It can also be used as a noticeboard, for example listing general reference material or attaching notices to metal-backed boards using magnets.

Whiteboards offer a very limited scope for preparing material as there is only one surface for recording information. However, you may want to plan how to use it to make 'spontaneous' notes and drawings during the session.

When using a whiteboard remember to:

- Check that all the students have a clear view of the board.

- Keep your handwriting clear and large enough to be seen from the back of the room.

- Erase material with a damp cloth or sponge when you have finished, otherwise it may distract your audience.

- Remember to use the correct (non-permanent) marker pens. (If you use the wrong pen you will need a cleaning agent to remove the marks.)

- Bring your own spare pens.

- Avoid obstructing the audience's view when writing on the board. If you are right-handed, stand with the board on your left side. Start writing or drawing about a third of the way in so your body is not obstructing the audience's view. If you are left-handed, stand with the board on your right side. Use the first two thirds of the board (the part furthest away from you).

### Flipchart

Flipcharts, like whiteboards, are very useful as notepads for workshop or seminar discussions. The sheets tear off, making them ideal for use in recording group discussions like brainstorms. Unlike the whiteboard the sheets can be retained for reference later in the seminar.

When using flipchart sheets remember to:

- Check that all the students have a clear view of the flipchart.

- Keep your handwriting clear and large enough to be seen from the back of the room.

- Use the flipchart for only brief periods, as you will have to turn away from the audience to do any writing.

- Cover any material when you have finished otherwise it may distract the audience. Either mask with paper or leave blank pages in between your prepared sheets.

- ○ Fold back sheets rather than tearing them off, as you may need to refer to them later.

- ○ Avoid obstructing the audience's view when using the flipchart. If you are right-handed, stand with the chart on your left side. Start writing or drawing about a third of the way in so your body is not obstructing the audience's view. If you are left-handed, stand with the chart on your right side. Use the first two thirds of the chart (the part furthest away from you).

- ○ Large flipcharts are difficult to transport but smaller, desktop varieties are available. These are handy for preparing material in advance, but their small size restricts their use to groups of ten or less.

### Handouts

Trainers and lecturers use handouts in numerous ways. Some are designed for use in preparing for a session, for example a list of preparatory reading or a document containing introductory material. Many are for use during the session, for example a gapped handout to be completed by the student during the lecture, while others are to promote further individual study by the student after the session, for example a reading list.

Use handouts to:

- ○ provide preparatory reading, for example background information, glossary of terms or 'stop and think' activities

- ○ provide complex information such as detailed numerical data or diagrams

- ○ give evidence in support of the main arguments, for example research studies, detailed case studies and explanations

- ○ aid note-taking by supplying copies of essential acetates or illustrations

- ○ encourage active listening by supplying gapped handouts to be completed during the lecture, for example labelling a diagram or filling in key terms

- ○ encourage self-assessment by using true/false or multiple-choice questionnaires

- o facilitate learning activities, for example instructions for practical tasks, data sets and case studies for problem solving
- o give students the opportunity to apply new concepts or principles, for example analysing data sets
- o promote further study by giving lists of references, further reading or a set of questions to focus students' reading and note-taking.

Preparation:

- o Remember to make the handout meaningful for the student. It is not there to impress. Think carefully about what you want it to achieve.
- o Explain terminology and limit the amount of unfamiliar information you use in preparatory reading.
- o Always review pre-course handouts at the start of the session. This will help to clear up any misunderstandings or confusions.
- o Make them user-friendly by organising information and taking care in presentation.

When using handouts remember to:

- o Decide on a system for distribution as giving out paper to a large group is time-consuming and may disrupt the flow of your presentation. Some ideas are to:
  - o Place handouts on chairs before the audience arrives.
  - o Leave handouts at the back of the room for people to collect as they leave.
  - o Ask the student representatives from the group to collect and distribute them before the session.
  - o Supply a small number to be held for reference in the library.
- o Always tell the audience what handouts you will be supplying, especially if they are expecting to take notes.

**Evaluation**

Monitor the cost-effectiveness and efficacy of your teaching materials. Ask yourself:

- What materials and equipment did I use?
- How much time was spent preparing materials?
- How much did they cost to produce?
- Did they achieve what I intended?
- Were they used at the planned point during the session?
- Could they have been used more effectively?
- Were they redundant?
- How were they interpreted? Was it in the way that I intended?
- What was the student feedback about teaching materials?

---

## Summary Points

- Additional written materials, such as acetates, slides, flipcharts or handouts, are used to support teaching.

- They add interest to a presentation and help maintain attention, memory and understanding.

- Decide on your teaching objectives, learning outcomes and content before you start to plan how you can use teaching materials.

- The purpose, cost and time required to prepare materials will all influence your choice.

- Match your materials to your students' needs.
- Make sure your text and visuals are legible.
- Use colour to add interest and help the audience understand information faster.
- Evaluate the development, use and effectiveness of your teaching materials.

# 9

# Teaching and Learning Skills in Context
## Note-taking

Note-taking is one of the core study skills that students need to master. Although notes are traditionally associated with lectures, students will be required to record information from a variety of sources. These will include books, journal articles, audiovisual material, demonstrations and the student's own clinical experience. In common with other skills it requires practice, and it is not as straightforward as it might seem at first.

This section reviews the purpose of note-taking, and looks at how study notes facilitate the learning process. It also offers students some practical suggestions on how to improve their skills in note-taking.

**Purpose of notes**

There are several reasons for taking notes as a student. They can be used as both a learning tool and as a study aid for revision.

Notes provide:

1.  A record

2.  A framework

3.  A reference source

4.  An aide-mémoire

5.  A learning tool

6.  A revision aid.

*1. A record*

Notes will provide a permanent record of your studies. They will contain information that will help you understand the theoretical background and practical applications of your subject. Good notes will also contain *your* thoughts, opinions and ideas, making them a true reflection of the development in your learning.

### 2. A framework
Your notes are a way to organise both your past and your current learning. They provide a framework that makes it easier to assimilate new information with what you have already learnt.

You will also be able to gauge how well you comprehend current studies. Gaps or sketchy notes indicate that further reading or more in-depth study is required.

### 3. A reference source
Notes contain information that will be of use to you in preparing essays. This may be data that can be included in your assignment, or it may be references to other sources. Reading through your notes may even inspire you about topics that you would like to study in more depth.

### 4. An aide-mémoire
Notes will help to remind you of facts, figures, theories and practical applications that would otherwise be forgotten. Their permanent and personal nature means that you will be able to return to them at any point – so you can find information you have collected from journal articles, books and audiovisual material without the need to seek out the original texts or tapes.

### 5. A learning tool
Notes are a way of organising information, which will help you make sense of what the lecturer or author is trying to convey. In good notes, the key information will be highlighted and clearly distinguished from supporting examples and explanations. The link between topics will be clear, and you will be able to see how smaller details fit into the whole picture.

### 6. A revision aid
Your notes as a whole will provide you with an overview of the areas around which to plan your revision. They can also be used to help you remember key facts and identify themes.

The actual task of note-taking itself is one way of starting to memorise the material. Rereading notes at regular intervals helps to consolidate the retention of this information.

**Note-taking skills**

Notes are personal to each student. They are not usually placed under external scrutiny, nor do they form part of any assessment. There is no direct system for evaluating the ability of a student to make relevant and useful notes. Of course, poor notes ultimately result in poor performance. However, this does not help students identify ways to improve their skills or how to make the most of the information they have recorded.

Some students are uncertain about which pieces of information they should be noting. In order not to miss anything they conscientiously record every utterance of the lecturer, or neatly précis a chapter or article. This results in over-detailed notes where it is difficult to identify the key points or get a perspective of the topic as a whole. It is also extremely tedious for the student and does not promote active listening or critical thought.

However, students need to be wary of making too brief a set of notes. This may miss out some of the key points and make it difficult to use the notes for revision.

The amount and type of information that needs to be recorded will vary between students. It depends very much on what individuals need in order to make sense of what is being presented to them.

**Different styles of note-taking**

Have you ever considered the way in which you record information? Most of us tend to follow the style of note-taking shown to us at school. The following section describes several different methods of note-taking.

***Sequential notes***

These notes are also known as outline or linear notes. They are the most traditional approach to note-taking, and the one most likely to have been modelled at school. Information is recorded in the same sequence in which it is given, thereby replicating the lecturer's or the author's organisation of the information. Key points and supporting evidence is recorded down the page. Headings, underlining, numbering or lettering systems are used to indicate the hierarchy and distinguish one topic from another. See Figure 9.1 for an example of sequential notes.

'Legislation and Record Keeping'

> **<u>Records</u>** – <u>documentation</u> might be:
>> **Primary**: casenote folders, admission sheets, referral letters, case history sheets, assessment information, progress notes, operation sheets, nursing careplans
>> **Secondary**: x-rays, drug sheets
>> **Transitory**: blood pressure charts, temperature charts

> **<u>Legislation</u>** –
>> **Common law**: e.g. 'The Bolam Test'
>> **Statutory law**: 'Acts' are enacted by parliament, e.g. 'The Data Protection Act 1998'

> <u>Relevant legislation</u>
>> The Data Protection Act 1998
>> Access to Health Records 1990 (deceased)

*Figure 9.1 Sequential notes*

*Advantages*

- ○ The hierarchical structure of the information is easy to see. (This of course depends on how logical the author or lecturer was in structuring the original material.)

- ○ If the notes are well spaced out then corrections and noting of additional information is easily made.

*Disadvantages*

- ○ Sequential note-taking is often a passive task that allows students to avoid interpreting and assimilating information for themselves.

- ○ The student is more likely to record information in the words of the lecturer and author, so there is a greater chance of unintentional plagiarism.

- ○ The 'whole picture' is harder to see as information is spread over several pages.

*Tips on using sequential notes effectively*

Avoid cramming the page with notes. Use A4 size paper and only write on one side of the paper. Set wide margins and leave spaces between lines and paragraphs. This way you can add extra information, note any questions you want to follow up or make an aide-mémoire to yourself.

The arrangement of your notes should convey the hierarchy of the information. Use headings, underlining and highlighting to help distinguish between a major point and the explanations and examples used to support it.

Put things of particular importance, like examples, quotes or references, in boxes.

It is not necessary to record information in grammatically correct sentences. Leave out any extraneous words, and get into the habit of using abbreviations.

### Spider web notes

The main theme of the lecture, book chapter or article is written in the middle of the page. The key points or topics that relate to this central idea are written in one- or two-word phrases and spaced around the page. Further details are noted around the relevant key point. Colour, lines and arrows are used to show how points link together and to indicate the hierarchy of the information. See Figure 9.2 for an example of spider web notes.

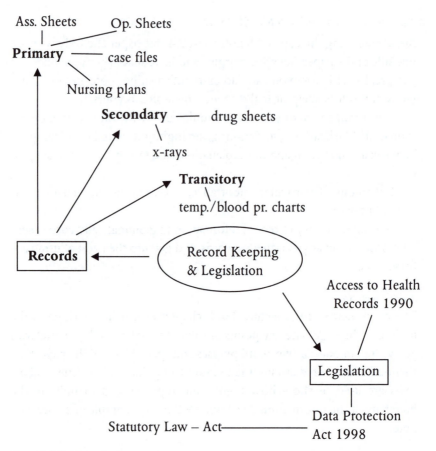

*Figure 9.2 Spider web notes*

*Advantages*

- ○ The student is required to make his or her own selection and interpretation of the data. This process aids learning and also encourages the student to put ideas into his or her own words.

- ○ The scope of the topic is clearly illustrated by the resulting diagram.

- ○ The breakdown of the topic into its constituent parts is clearly visible.

*Disadvantages*

- ○ Errors are difficult to amend.
- ○ You are restricted to recording information on one page.
- ○ It is difficult to include large diagrams, definitions, quotes and so on.
- ○ The original order of the material is lost.

*Tips on using spider web notes effectively*

Space the main subtopics out around the page, so you have enough room to add in minor details.

Use different styles of arrows to indicate different relationships between topics.

Use colour to distinguish between different levels of information – so the central idea would be in one colour, all the subtopics in another, and a third colour used for all the supporting details. (Highlighter pens are a quick and easy method.)

Alternatively use different shapes to outline words and phrases – so the central idea is in a square, the subtopics in a squiggly circle, and the minor details in a simple circle.

Use pictures and symbols as well as words to represent key ideas.

**Pattern notes**

These are similar to spider web notes, with the core theme or idea written in the centre of the page (Taylor 1992). However, lines are drawn radiating out from the centre to key points. Supporting details or a further breakdown of the topic is listed alongside the relevant line. See Figure 9.3 for an example of pattern notes.

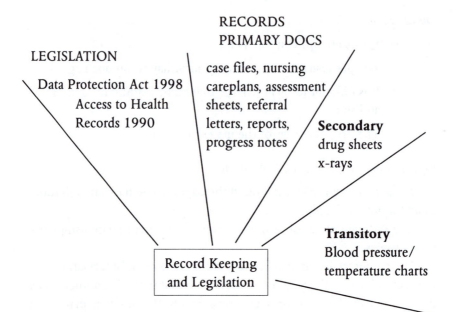

*Figure 9.3 Pattern notes*

*Advantages*

- ○ The student is required to make his or her own selection and interpretation of the data. This process aids learning and also encourages the student to put ideas into his or her own words.

- ○ It provides a useful summary of the topic for revision.

*Disadvantages*

- ○ It is only possible to record a limited amount of information.
- ○ The original organisation of the material is lost.
- ○ It is difficult to organise unfamiliar material.

*Tips on using pattern notes effectively*

Use the whole of the page for your diagram. Allow plenty of space between the radiating lines to add in detail.

Be concise and use keywords only.

Use colour or different styles of lettering to differentiate between main topics and subtopics.

## Note-taking in different contexts

### Lectures

You will be more able to cope with new information if you have done some preparation before your lecture. Make sure you know how and where the lecture fits into your course outline, and complete any recommended preparatory reading. This includes making time to reread notes from any previous lectures or related clinical experience.

Think of some questions that you would like answered by the lecturer. This is more likely to help you focus your attention by making you an active participant rather than a passive recipient of information. Alternatively you can try some lateral thinking during the class by writing the questions you think the lecturer is trying to answer in his or her talk.

As stated above it is not a good idea to try to write down everything that you hear or copy every diagram and drawing. It is very unlikely that you will be able to keep up with the pace of the lecturer, and it is difficult to listen at the same time as you are writing. You must therefore make decisions about which pieces of information to note.

Burnett (1979) reminds us that it is the 'point', not just the words, that needs to be recorded. This is a useful observation to bear in mind when making notes. What point or message do you think the lecturer is attempting to communicate?

The lecturer will often help you by giving verbal and non-verbal cues about the importance of an item and how topics link together. Listen out for prompt phrases that signal a main point, for example, 'this is the key concept' or 'there are three principles'. Key points are often listed on overheads or reiterated in handouts. Other phrases, like 'in contrast' or 'similarly', tell you about the connection between ideas. Non-verbal cues will also give you information; for example, speakers often pause before an important point.

Make a conscious selection from the explanations, examples and references used to support the lecturer's main arguments. Which ones are of most use to you? Thinking of your own examples is one way to help make sense of the information.

Set aside 20 minutes to review your notes as soon as possible after the end of the lecture. Reread them and check for accuracy. This task is often more usefully done in conjunction with another student or in a study group. Check you have all the main points and look out for any information you have omitted or were unclear about. Try to fill in the gaps or identify where you can follow up information. This may be in a tutorial or a reading session, or you may need to go back to the lecturer.

### Written material

Before making any notes think carefully about your purpose in reading the material. What questions would you like answered? Are there any specific facts and figures that you want to find out? This will help you in only noting the details relevant for your task, rather than spending time in writing a précis of the whole article or chapter. (See Chapter 7 for more information on 'effective reading'.)

It may be necessary to record some information word for word. This includes dates, names, references to further reading, quotes and definitions. You may also want to copy diagrams and drawings. However, in written material it may be quicker to photocopy reference lists and detailed illustrations. See 'How does the copyright law affect photocopying' in Chapter 19.

Start to compile a bibliography by recording the books and articles you have used for your notes. Record the information either manually using a card index or electronically on a computer database. Each method has its own advantages. Index cards are cheap, portable and easy to use. Notes can be quickly scribbled down as you browse through the shelves at the library. However, if you need to compile a reference list, then a database is the preferred method. See Chapter 17, 'Getting the Best Out of Your Personal Computer', for more information on databases.

Make sure you record all the information required to fulfil your institution's guidelines on writing references. See Chapter 12, 'Dissertations', for more information about writing references. The following details are usually recorded.

For books:

- title
- author(s) (including first names)
- year of publication
- edition
- publisher
- place of publication
- library and classification number

- o précis of content
- o personal notes on usefulness, readability.

For articles:

- o title
- o author(s) (including first names)
- o year of publication
- o journal title
- o journal volume/issue number
- o pages containing article
- o library and shelf number or topic code.

Make brief notes on articles and store these by subject headings.

### Practical demonstrations

Keep note-taking to a minimum in any sort of practical demonstration. The emphasis will be on showing you what is happening, and in some cases on you joining in and having a go yourself. It is difficult to combine this sort of practical experience with note-taking. If you do get a chance to jot something down, then follow these rules:

1. Make a note of what you *see* and *hear.*

2. Record any information you think you are unlikely to find in a textbook or lecture.

3. Write down technical terms and check them out later.

4. Write up your thoughts as soon as possible after the demonstration.

### Organising your notes

Sort and file your notes immediately, otherwise they will build up into a mound of paperwork that will be frustrating and of little use to your studies. Think about how you want to organise and store your notes. The system you choose must be flexible, allow easy retrieval of information and be practical to use.

The most common and probably the best method is to file loose-leaf sheets in A4 size ring binders. These binders allow you to insert additional notes where you want them, as well as having the capacity to hold a large amount of paper.

Find a place to store your ring binders that is easily accessible. If you lack the space or funds for a set of shelves, a cheap alternative is to use cardboard boxes from your local supermarket. These should be medium-sized with stout sides and base. Place the box on its side so that the ring binders can be filed in an upright position. Box files can be stored upright or horizontally. You now have a ready-made shelving unit. The box is easily carried by the precut handgrips for storage out of the way in a cupboard.

Decide how you want to file information. Your system needs to be logical, adaptable and easy to cross-reference. Avoid having to access several different files to get the required information. Notes can be arranged by subject or discipline. You may want to separate theoretical modules from clinical experience, or you may want to integrate the two. Choose a categorisation system that allows you to quickly locate the information you need to prepare for essays and revise for assessments.

You will need to devise a cataloguing system as soon as you start your note-taking. Use dividers to sort information into more manageable sections. Label each file and keep a list of contents at the beginning. Make an index that covers all of your files, and update it regularly.

Journals, newspapers cuttings and other resource materials are best stored in box files. These should be catalogued in the same way as your ring binders. Make a note of any cross-references between your resource materials and your filed notes. You can also use colour coding to organise files, for example so that your box file is the same colour as its related ring binder.

Clearly mark each set of notes with information that will identify its source. For lectures, this will be the title, name and designation of the lecturer, along with the date. It might also be useful to make a note of the module under which the lecture was scheduled. Notes taken from articles, books or audiovisual material need to have sufficient information to allow you to locate the original material at a later date.

## Review

Regularly review your notes. Are there any areas that need expanding? Do you have enough examples or supporting evidence? Follow up references and make notes from any handouts. Are you unclear about any aspects? Write these as questions and find out by reading or talking with peers or lecturers.

Keep your notes dynamic by regularly updating them. Assimilate information gleaned from other sources into your lecture notes at the appropriate place. For example, notes from clinical practice, where you have seen a chronic asthmatic, might be filed along with your lecture notes on respiratory diseases. This helps continuity by placing information in context.

## Action Points

1. Practise your note-taking skills. Make notes on a radio or television programme. Start with programmes that give simple, straightforward advice, then try documentaries and debates that give opposing arguments.

   Try to record these programmes so you can compare the information contained in your notes with the original source. Are your notes accurate? Did you leave out any important points or evidence?

2. Use different note-taking styles to record information from the same programme. Which style do you prefer? What method made you think more about what you were writing down? How do the different sets of notes compare – do they each contain the same key points and examples? Which notes would you like to use for revision purposes? Which notes are suitable for preparing an essay?

3. Work with other students in a pair or a small group. Compare notes on a lecture or article. Did everybody record the same information? Is there agreement on the key points? Are there any items the group wants to follow up? Discuss any questions that the group felt were still unanswered.

4. The above material can be used to discuss different styles of note-taking. Look at how each student has noted the information. List what the group thinks is helpful about each method. Are there any disadvantages?

5. Share your ideas about improving your note-taking skills with a friend. Each person makes a list of two things about his or her note-taking that are good, and two things he or she would like to improve. Talk about your list with your friend, and set a date when you think you will have achieved them. Arrange to

meet up again to check out your lists. Your list might include things like improving accuracy, filing notes and keeping your index up to date or trying a different way of recording information.

6.  Your notes are useful for revision. Regularly reading through them will help you remember information and improve your understanding. Try to actively recall the main points or summaries at regular intervals.

---

### Summary Points

- Notes are both a learning tool and a study aid for revision.
- There are several different styles of note-taking that include sequential notes, spider web notes and pattern notes.
- Good note-taking requires preparation.
- Make your listening or reading active by thinking of questions you would like answered by the lecture, book or demonstration.
- Record the point of a lecture, written material or demonstration, not just the words.
- Keep your notes organised with an index and regularly update and review.

# 10

# Essays

Training courses for health professionals usually require students to write at least one essay, if not several, as part of the assessment process. These assignments demand an enormous amount of time and effort from both the student and the examiner. However, they are essential in helping tutors gauge the level of each individual's performance.

Essays provide students with the opportunity to demonstrate to the tutor their ability to:

- recall the pertinent facts of a subject
- select and organise information
- understand the relationship between ideas
- express ideas in a coherent and logical manner
- formulate opinions and convey convincing arguments to support their views
- discuss the practical application of theories.

As well as demonstrating these abilities to their tutor, it will also give the students feedback on how well they understand the subject. This can help them in refining personal learning goals.

As well as being part of the assessment process, the task of preparing and formulating essays is in itself a learning process. First, the obligation to write such papers is a useful catalyst in encouraging them to read more broadly and in depth about the subject matter in question. This research is always necessary to supplement lectures and tutorials. Second, the students' thinking about the subject is developed through the process of selecting and organising information into a cohesive account. Studying in this way aids the retention of information for use in formal examinations and, more importantly, in clinical practice.

Some students have had little experience of essay writing before they start their training. Other students, who may have returned to education after working for several years, may feel they need to revise their composition skills. If this applies to you, the following section gives advice on how to plan, write and understand the assessment of essays.

### Planning

A good essay requires a good plan. It will help you to:

- understand the breadth and depth of the task
- refine your research task
- organise your notes
- select information relevant to your essay title
- structure your essay.

Stages in the planning process are:

1. Establishing the terms of reference

2. Analysing the essay title

3. Writing an outline.

### 1. Establishing the terms of reference

Find out from your tutor any specific instructions regarding your set essay. These are likely to be about:

- The length of the essay. What is the minimum and maximum number of words?

- The content of the essay. Have you been asked to include examples from clinical practice? Is it purely about theory? Do you have to relate theory to practice?

- The sources for the essay. Is there a list of directed reading? Are you required to provide references to recent research?

- The timeframe. What are your deadlines?

- Presentation. What are the guidelines about the format in which the essay must be submitted?

- Assessment criteria. Is information available on how marks are allocated?

### 2. Analysing the essay title

Always start by reading the title very carefully. Any mistakes in your interpretation of the assignment will lose you marks or might even cause you to fail.

Essay titles are phrased as questions, instructions, or statements on which you will be asked to comment. Start by identifying the main components of the title by underlining all the keywords. These words will tell you both the topic and the approach your tutor wants you to take in the essay.

For example:

> Outline the principles of the Data Protection Act (1998) and give examples of how these can be applied to record keeping in a community setting.

You can now decide which of the keywords tells you 'what' or 'who' is the subject of the essay.

> Outline the principles of the Data Protection Act (1998) and give examples of how these can be applied to record keeping in a community setting.

The main subject matter is 'the Data Protection Act (1998)'.

Look at the question again and see how the examiner has further defined the subject area by asking for the '*principles*'. The question is not asking for information about the background to the Act or how it is enforced.

Each subject area will have a wealth of information that would be far too much to include in one essay. Therefore, questions usually set one or more parameters within which you must restrict your answer. These often refer to:

- time periods, for example, 'since the 1940s', 'in the twentieth century', 'in the last decade'

- specific regions or nations, for example, 'European', 'in the Third World', 'inner city'

- ○ specific sectors of the health service, for example, 'community care', 'hospice' and 'acute'
- ○ specific aspects of health care, for example, 'record keeping', 'moving a client' or 'type of therapy'.

The parameters will help you to identify what is of relevance and importance to include in your answer. In the above example, you are asked about 'record keeping' in a 'community setting'.

The keywords left in the question will be the ones that ask or command you to do something. These will be verbs like 'define', 'analyse', 'discuss' or 'compare and contrast'.

The directions tell you what you have to do with your information, and there are two main types – descriptive and analytical (Leader 1990).

Essay titles that request a descriptive answer focus on testing your knowledge of the facts and figures. They are likely to include one of the following directions:

- ○ Describe = give a detailed account.
- ○ Define = give the meaning of, describe exactly, make clear the limits of a subject or issue.
- ○ Outline = provide an overview of the main points.
- ○ Illustrate or show how = use explanations, examples, analogies, diagrams and drawings.

Analytical essay titles require you to show a deeper level of understanding. You must be able to not only recall facts and figures, but also to make judgements and evaluate the information. They are likely to include one of the following directions:

- ○ Assess = weigh up alternative arguments or viewpoints.
- ○ Evaluate or judge = determine the worth or value of something.
- ○ Account for or explain = give reasons, provide evidence.
- ○ Compare and contrast = describe similarities and differences.
- ○ Compare = emphasis is on the similarities between items.
- ○ Contrast or differentiate or distinguish = emphasis is on the differences between items.
- ○ Explore or examine or investigate = ask questions about, scrutinise evidence carefully.

- Criticise = give arguments for and against, examine good and bad points.
- Discuss = evaluate different viewpoints.
- Analyse = study in detail, divide into component parts.
- Apply = relate one set of knowledge to another set or different context; usually asks for a practical application.

In the above example the examiner is asking the student first to *outline* or provide an overview of the main principles, then second to give *examples* that show how it can be *applied* to record keeping in the community setting.

### 3. Writing an outline

Your analysis of the title will lead you to start formulating a general plan or outline for your essay. The most common method is to brainstorm your thoughts and ideas about the subject matter that you have identified in the essay question.

If you have difficulty in thinking up ideas, it may be necessary to do some background reading first. This will give you a general impression of the subject and will help you in identifying some key points. However, delay starting any in-depth research until you have your initial outline. Unless you have a clear-cut plan there is a danger of spending a disproportionate amount of time on one area that you later find is irrelevant to your essay.

It may help to set a series of questions about a key concept, topic or word (Newman 1989) – So you might ask the following questions about the Data Protection Act (1998):

- What is an 'Act'?
- What is meant by 'data'?
- How does it 'protect'?
- Who does it apply to?
- Why was it introduced?

This will help you identify the areas for your research.

Once you have completed your brainstorm you can start to identify the main points and group related ideas together. You are now ready to think about how you will organise this information. There are various ways of structuring your essay (see below in 'Writing Your Essay' for more information). In our example the outline might look something like this:

## Introduction

What is an 'Act'?

What is the purpose of the Data Protection Act (1998)?

Brief reference to link with Data Protection Act (1984).

Who or what does the Act apply to?

Explain introducing principles along with examples.

## Main part

- ○ Data processed fairly and lawfully
  – confidentiality
  (e.g. security systems for data held on computer; protecting confidentiality for clients where records are held in the home)

- ○ Purpose for processing information
  (e.g. client consent to process information; clinician informing client how information will be used)

- ○ Protection of information
  (e.g. secure storage; destruction of records)

- ○ Access
  (e.g. client-held records; retention of records for minimum periods)

- ○ Data to be:
  - ○ relevant
  - ○ accurate
  - ○ up to date
  - ○ not excessive

(e.g. record keeping guidelines for clinicians; recording notes contemporaneously).

## Conclusion

Reiterate main principle that data must be processed fairly and lawfully.

Sum up main points.

Use your outline to help in organising the information you collect through reading, seminars and lectures, for example filing notes under confidentiality, use of information, Data Protection Act (1998) and so on. This will help when you start to write your essay as all the information for each section will already be collated.

You will find that your outline will change as you find out more about the subject and develop your ideas. Some details may be discarded or new information added in. Try out different outlines until you find the best structure for your essay.

Start at an early stage to think about the allocation of words within your essay. Some sections might need to be longer as the points are more important or relate to a broader issue. Some may be minor and therefore require fewer words. Planning in this way will keep you on track and help you balance out the essay content.

Remember that without a clear plan your essay is likely to:

- lack structure
- contain irrelevant material
- omit important facts
- have an imbalance in the content
- fall short of or exceed the word limit.

Once the title has been analysed and the outline drawn up you will have important clues about:

- what topics to research
- what type of information:
  - knowledge
  - skills
  - statistics
  - principles
  - policies
  - legislation
  - clinical guidelines
  - clinical experience
  - clinical roles and responsibilities

- what information is relevant to the essay
- how to structure the essay
- how to present the information.

## Research

Always take time to constantly refer back to your analysis of the title and your outline when researching your essay. See Chapter 7 'Writing As an Aid to Learning' for more information on how to search for information.

## Writing your essay

Essays consist of a three part structure:

1. The introduction
2. The main section
3. The conclusion.

### 1. The introduction

All essays need some form of introduction to set the scene for the reader. It will briefly state:

- what you are about to tell the reader
- why you are going to tell this to the reader
- how you will tell it.

In other words, the introduction lets your reader know the (a) content, (b) rationale and (c) structure of your essay.

### (a) Content

Your introduction will give your readers an idea of the key points or issues to be discussed in your essay. They will then have a framework that will help them to organise and make sense of the information as they read through the rest of the essay. By being able to select the important details, you will also show the examiner that you have understood the question.

Some topics may necessitate a brief overview of the background or history of the subject in order to place your discussion in context. Remember to keep this to a short summary that contains only the essential points, otherwise you may get sidetracked into giving an overlong account of something that is minor to your overall argument. This will result in an unbalanced account and may mean you are unable to cover the relevant material in enough detail.

Use references in your introduction if appropriate. This will help set the tone of your essay by indicating that you have thoroughly researched your topic. However, do not be tempted to write a paragraph that merely contains a series of quotes. References are there to support your views and not replace them. The examiner will want to read your thoughts and opinions on the subject.

### (b) Rationale

You may also use the introduction to explain your approach to the subject matter and how you have interpreted the question, for example the particular aspects of the problem you will focus on and why you have taken this perspective.

### (c) Structure

Giving your reader details of how the essay is structured will help to orientate them. For instance, you may need to describe x in order to understand how y relates to z. They will then understand when you start with a description of x before discussing the relationship between y and z.

The introduction forms approximately 12 per cent of your essay – so in a 2000 word composition you would plan to have an introduction of about 250 words.

Pitfalls to avoid:

- Writing an overlong introduction so that the essay becomes unbalanced.

- Repeating the title either verbatim or only slightly adapted as the opening paragraph to your essay.

- Opting out of writing an introduction by replacing it with a quote, analogy or definition. These devices are not meant to stand alone.

- Being unoriginal and copying another student's ideas on the introduction – especially if the idea to start with a standard quote is being used by several students. This is very boring for the marker and not the best way to impress him or her!

- Starting to write the main body of the essay in the introduction.

  ○  Writing a conclusion and not an introduction.

  ○  Writing an introduction that bears no relation to the question
     or what you are about to say in the rest of the essay.

### 2. The main section

The main or middle part will come after your introduction and will form
the bulk of your essay. It is here that you will demonstrate to the marker
your knowledge and understanding of the subject matter.

*Structure*

There are different ways to organise the information in your essay. Your
choice of structure will depend on the subject matter and the requirements
given in the title. Here are some examples:

(a) 'Illustrate what is meant by the "use and
      protection" of information within the NHS.'

    several themes                    (use and protection of
                                      client information)

    theme one (confidentiality)

    theme two (access to records)

    theme three (use of information)


(b) 'Discuss the role of the clinician in ensuring client
     confidentiality.'

    one theme (confidentiality)

    general infomation (definition, rights to, duty of confidentiality)

         specific information on role of:

    processing information        access              storage

(c) 'Distinguish between language delay and language disorder.'


| delay<br>disorder | Theme one<br>(pattern of development) |

| delay<br>disorder | Theme two<br>(response to therapy) |

| delay<br>disorder | Theme three<br>(communication styles) |

OR

| Language delay | Theme one – pattern of development<br>Theme two – response to therapy<br>Theme three – communication styles |

| Language disorder | Theme one – pattern of development<br>Theme two – response to therapy<br>Theme three – communication styles |

As you can see from the above there are numerous ways to structure your essay. The main criterion is that you cluster information to help the reader make connections between ideas. The sequence in which you present these clusters must be logical and coherent. Is there a logical progression in your argument? Does one point lead clearly on to another?

*Content*

Use your analysis of the title and your outline to help you judge whether your choice of material is relevant to the question. Think about whether it is a primary point, secondary point or supporting evidence, such as an example or reference to another source. If you can omit some data without making a difference to your overall argument or discussion then it is likely that it is redundant.

Constantly check back with your original plan to make sure you remain true to the question. Check that you have answered the question as it has been asked. For example, has your answer changed from 'why does x cause z' to 'what causes z'?

Your tutor will be looking for an expression of your point of view; however, you must support this with evidence from the literature. Make sure that you have read widely before attempting the essay. You will then be able to discuss a range of theories and refer to information from a number of sources. Remember to acknowledge these both in the text and by supplying a reference list at the end of the essay.

The main part forms approximately 75 to 80 per cent of your essay – so in a 2000 word composition you would plan to use 1500 words for the main part of the essay.

Pitfalls to avoid:

- Showing a bias by the type of information you select or the viewpoint you put across.
- Using too much of the essay to write about one or two points so that you have to skim over the others.
- Omiting key information.
- Not bothering with a structure so that your writing is confused and jumps back and forth between different points.
- Failing to do any background reading so that your essay presents a very narrow viewpoint.

### 3. The conclusion

The conclusion helps to draw your essay to a close. It will contain either a summary of the key points, a statement of the outcome of your discussion or a resolution to your argument. Making a reference back to your introduction or the original question brings the essay full circle and achieves a satisfactory closure.

Some questions that might help you in writing your conclusion are:

- What are the main points of your essay?
- Is there a theme that links these main points?
- How will your essay have changed a naïve reader?

- a change in attitude
- a change in knowledge
- a change in how to apply theory to practice
- a change in awareness
- a change in understanding.
  - What general application has the information in your essay?
    - to improve practice
    - to indicate areas for further research
    - to highlight a debate or controversy.

Pitfalls to avoid

- Writing an overlong conclusion.
- Ending the essay abruptly and failing to draw together the main points.
- Including new information, an additional argument or viewpoint not mentioned in the rest of the essay.
- Writing a conclusion that bears no relation to the question or what you have said in the rest of the essay.

Like the introduction, the conclusion forms about 12 per cent of your essay – so in a 2000 word composition you would plan to have a conclusion of about 250 words.

### Writing drafts

Views are mixed about whether writing several drafts is a good idea or not. Some advise writing coursework essays under exam conditions as practice for timed examinations. This may help in preparing you for your exams, however it is unlikely to help you in producing your best piece of work. I would recommend that, like any other written task, you take the opportunity to draft your essay and revise it as necessary before you submit it. Use the checklist in the 'Action Points' at the end of this chapter to help edit your draft.

### Assessment criteria

There is no set marking scheme that is used as a standard by all tutors for assessing essays. The way in which this type of written work is assessed varies between markers and between institutions. It will also depend on the type of essay to be marked.

Some tutors work out a system where a set amount of marks is awarded to each main point covered in the essay. The accumulated figure is then converted into a percentage, which in turn may be used to place the student within a band or grade. This tends to work well with descriptive questions, but is less useful for essays where a greater depth of understanding needs to be demonstrated by the student.

Analytical questions benefit from an approach where assessment is based on a variety of criteria that reflect several subsets of skills. The features of an essay commonly assessed using this method are:

1.  Knowledge of the subject

2.  Understanding of the subject

3.  Writing skills

4.  Essay skills

5.  Style

6.  Presentation.

The marker will be looking for evidence of the student's performance in each of these skill areas.

### 1. Knowledge of the subject

- Evidence –

    - Able to recall facts and figures accurately.

- Breadth of knowledge base
  Evidence –

    - All key points are covered.

    - Evidence of extensive reading.

- Depth of knowledge base
  Evidence –

    - Demonstrates a detailed knowledge of facts and figures.

    - Able to describe theories involving more abstract concepts, models and processes.

## 2. Understanding of the subject

- Ability to analyse information
  Evidence –
  - Able to identify key components of an idea or concept.
  - Able to problem-solve.
  - Recognises patterns and relationships.
- Ability to select relevant material
  Evidence –
  - Good choice of specific issues to illustrate general points.
  - Quotes and examples used with a clear purpose.
- Ability to evaluate
  Evidence –
  - Able to critically appraise – gives pros and cons.
  - Shows recognition of controversies.
  - Recognises significance of information.
- Ability to apply
  Evidence –
  - Gives examples of how to apply knowledge.

## 3. Writing skills

- Evidence –
  - Text is readable and interesting.
  - The message is expressed clearly.
  - Phrasing is concise without needless repetition.

## 4. Essay skills

- Interpretation
  Evidence –
  - Identified key elements of the title.
  - Structure and content of the essay complies with the requirements given in the title.

- ○ Research skills
  Evidence –
  - ○ Sources are acknowledged.
  - ○ A reference list is provided.
  - ○ Personal thoughts and ideas are supported with evidence from the literature.
- ○ Organisation of information
  Evidence –
  - ○ Essay has an identifiable structure.
  - ○ Information is organised into a logical sequence.
- ○ Content
  Evidence –
  - ○ Content is balanced.
  - ○ Subject matter limited in an appropriate way.

### 5. Style

- ○ Evidence –
  - ○ Student takes an original approach.
  - ○ Written in student's own words.
  - ○ Student's own ideas and thoughts are integrated into the whole.

### 6. Presentation

- ○ Evidence –
  - ○ Complied with guidelines.
  - ○ Spelling and grammar are correct.

Marking schemes are devised in a way that helps the tutor allocate marks according to the degree that the student has met the criteria. For example:

*Knowledge*

| detailed | 5 | 4 | 3 | 2 | 1 | sketchy |
| in-depth | 5 | 4 | 3 | 2 | 1 | shallow |
| thorough | 5 | 4 | 3 | 2 | 1 | superficial |

Tutors may use a weighting system so that certain skill subsets receive a higher percentage of the marks.

**Submitting your essay**

Ask your tutor or refer to your institutional guidelines about presentation and submission of your essay. It is vital that you comply with these otherwise you may lose marks or have your essay rejected.

In general essays must be:

- Typed – most institutions require essays to be either typed or word-processed on one side of good quality A4 paper.

- Well spaced – make sure you have adequate margins. The left-hand margin needs to be wider to allow for binding.

- Easy to read – keep lines well spaced and use a font size of at least 12 points.

- Easily marked – adequate margins and wide spacing provide space for the marker to write comments. Leave space at the end or add a blank sheet for the marker to put your grade and sum up his or her views.

- Paginated – number all pages except the front sheet.

- In order – put a front sheet at the beginning with:
  - the essay title
  - word length
  - your name
  - your tutor's name
  - the title of your course or learning unit
  - date of submission.

File diagrams, tables and so on near the page containing the relevant text.

Include a reference list at the end on a separate page.

  ○ Bound – place your essay in a folder that allows the pages to be easily turned and lies flat when opened. Remember to keep a copy for yourself.

## Action Points

1. Use the following checklist to help you edit the draft of your essay.

### *The structure of your essay*

❑ Your introduction is brief and states the what, why and how?

❑ You have covered all the main points.

❑ You have completed everything the title requires.

❑ Your answer remains true to what the question is asking.

❑ Your conclusion is brief with either a summary of the main points or your concluding arguments.

### *The content of your essay*

❑ There is a balance in what you have presented.

❑ You have only included information that is relevant to the title.

❑ Your presentation of the facts is unbiased.

❑ You have made links between ideas, and have analysed and interpreted the data where necessary.

❑ You have provided evidence to support your views and arguments.

❑ You have used quotes, examples, tables and diagrams to explain your ideas.

❑ Your figures, tables and quotes are accurate.

❑ You have made explicit the link between quotations or examples and your ideas and arguments.

*Your writing style*

- ❑ You make your points clearly.
- ❑ You have reduced unnecessary repetition.
- ❑ You have eliminated ambiguous wording.
- ❑ There is a logical development of ideas.

*You have indicated the sources for your essay*

- ❑ Your sources are cited in the text.
- ❑ A reference list is provided at the end of the essay.
- ❑ References cited in the text agree with those in the reference list.
- ❑ The style of referencing conforms with guidelines.

*You have complied with the terms of reference*

- ❑ Length is within the word limit.
- ❑ Spelling and grammar are correct.
- ❑ Page layout, style and binding conform with guidelines.

---

## Summary Points

- ° Essays are a means for tutors to gauge the level of individual students' performance.

- ° The task of preparing and formulating essays is also a learning process for the student.

- ° Before you start writing your essay, find out any specific instructions regarding length, content, directed reading, timeframe and presentation.

- ° Identify the keywords in the title. These will tell you both the topic and the approach you need to take in writing the essay.

- Use your analysis to formulate a plan or outline for your essay.

- Essays consist of a three part structure – an introduction, a main section and a conclusion.

- The introduction will tell the reader the content, structure and rationale for your approach.

- The structure of the main part of your essay will vary according to the subject and the requirements given in the title.

- The content needs to be relevant, balanced and unbiased and make reference to the literature.

- The conclusion will contain either a summary of the key points, a statement of the outcome of your discussion or a resolution to your argument.

- Drafting and editing your work several times will help you in producing your best piece of work.

- Assessment is usually based on a variety of criteria that reflect several subsets of skills.

- Always comply with your institution's guidelines about presentation and submission.

# 11

# Assessment

Most training courses have some form of summative assessment, either at the end of a study unit, term or academic year. This varies from multiple-choice and short answer to essay questions. Although students will know the structure of the assessment, the specific content of the exam paper is unseen. Unlike coursework these assessments are sat under exam conditions within a specified time period and invigilators are present to ensure that the regulations are met. An identical exam paper is used to assess students who are at the same point in their studies as parity in assessment is imperative.

Summative assessments help tutors in evaluating the student's level of knowledge and ability. A grade is assigned to the student's exam paper and indicates the level the student has attained. This is used in judging whether a professional qualification is awarded or not and to denote various degrees of achievement. These professional qualifications are seen as important indicators of competence by the general public, and are essential in establishing credibility for the health professional.

Preparation is the key to achieving a good standard of written work under exam conditions. There are three ways to prepare:

1. Be informed

2. Revise

3. Practise.

## 1. Be informed

In order to prepare efficiently, you need to know how and when you will be assessed. Find out as early as possible about the type of assessments you will be required to sit. Information about this is usually provided in your student handbook and past papers are held in the library.

Look at the structure of the paper – how many questions are there? Is it divided into sections? Is there a choice of questions? Are any questions compulsory? If there is a choice, are there any stipulations about this – for example, answer two from one section, one from another. It is essential that you are familiar with the structure of your paper before examination day.

## 2. Revise

Students worry about being able to recall information under the pressures of exam conditions where they are separated from their books and notes. Consistent and regular revision of notes helps in learning and memorising information.

Reading, reviewing notes and discussion help to consolidate and develop the student's understanding. This type of study immediately following a lecture also helps students remember information. It is estimated that students only remember half of what they hear in lectures if no active use is made of the material (Gibbs 1981).

Take steps to make your learning more active. Discuss with a peer:

- A problem from clinical practice. Will the information in the lecture or from your studies help to solve it?

- Your observations of a client. What in your notes will help you understand the behaviours you have observed?

- The type of information you would write in a leaflet for clients. What facts and figures that were provided in the lecture would you include?

- How ideas can be applied to clinical practice.

- Any statements or opinions you felt were provocative.

- The key points of the lecture.

One technique for helping in recall of information is the use of mind maps. This is an idea developed by Tony Buzan that helps not only memory but also the student's understanding of a topic. You start by placing the central theme, topic or keyword in the centre of the page. Buzan (1989) suggests that you use an image rather than a word, as this is more evocative and therefore memorable. The student then generates keywords and phrases around this central image using a brainstorming approach. Again pictures and symbols may be used to represent ideas rather than words.

Look at the example of a mind map about computers in Figure 11.1.

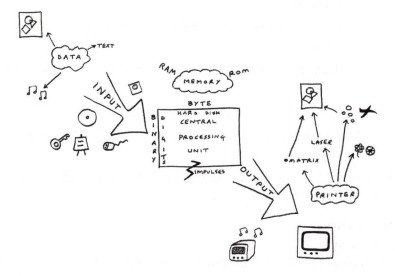

*Figure 11.1 A mind map*

See how related information has been grouped together on the page and arrows used to indicate the relationship between ideas.

The use of pictures rather than words for many items makes use of 'visualisation'. This is a memorisation technique where a picture is associated with a word or idea in order to aid recall.

Use mind maps to help you understand your revision notes and aid recall of information.

### 3. Practise

Summative assessments have to be completed within a set time period. This presents a challenge to most students regardless of their ability – so start to practise this skill early on in your course.

You can do this either individually or with a small peer group. Start by using plans or mind maps you have already generated to write out a full answer. Plan your timing for each section of your essay, and then compare this with the time it actually takes you in your practice session.

If you are consistently going over time, you need to identify ways of speeding up:

- Can you be more concise in the way that you express yourself?

- Have you included some information that is not relevant to the answer?

- Are you spending too much time thinking about how to say something?

- Is your plan or mind map clear enough?

- Do you know the information well enough so that recall is more automatic?

Work towards analysing the title, drafting a plan and writing an answer within the set time period.

## In the exam

### Read the paper

Take time to read through the questions on your paper at the start of the exam. Failure to comply with these directions is likely to lead to a reduced grade or a fail. For example, a fellow student failed an exam when he answered all five questions from the paper. In fact he only had to answer three. He had less time to answer each question and lost the chance to choose the best ones for him. An examiner in this situation will only mark the first three questions on the student's paper. If a compulsory question was omitted then a fail would be guaranteed.

### Make a choice

Choose the best questions for you. Ask yourself:

- Do I know all the facts and figures for this answer?

- Am I confident I understand the subject matter?

- Can I do what the question is asking (for example, you may be able to describe the what but not the why)?

- Am I able to limit my answer in an appropriate way (for example, it may be difficult to extract relevant information from a complicated subject)?

- What is the likely allocation of marks for my essay? Some questions combine a descriptive question with an analytical one. (See Chapter 10 'Essays' for further explanation of these types.) The descriptive part is likely to command fewer marks than the more complex analytical question. Plan your time and writing accordingly.

### Write a plan

Always make a rough plan on how you will answer the question. Aim to spend five to ten minutes on this task. This may seem excessive and a waste of your precious writing time. In fact a good plan will save you time and will make sure that you:

- understand what the question is asking
- plan your time effectively
- remember to include all the key points
- have a clear structure
- save on thinking time later, allowing you to just write your answer.

### Demonstrate your knowledge

Writing coursework will have helped prepare you for answering essay questions in an exam. The approach and execution is very similar. You will still be expected to demonstrate to the examiner the extent of your reading about the subject matter. This will partly be apparent from the range of views and theories you are able to discuss. It will also be demonstrated by your reference to other sources in your answer. Acknowledge these sources using names and dates where possible. You are not usually expected to give a reference list at the end of your answer.

### Write clearly

Exams are handwritten and as students are under pressure to complete the answers as quickly as possible, legibility often suffers. If you have large handwriting then write on every other line. Although you should not slow yourself down by trying to write as neatly as possible, it is still important that the marker can decipher your scribbles. Someone marking around 200 papers will not want to spend ten minutes trying to work out individual letters and words. Illegible work is likely to be unmarked, meaning you will lose precious points.

### Review

Leave time at the end to read back through your answer. You may want to add in a vital piece of information. Astute editing will also help improve the quality and accuracy of your work.

### Emergency solutions

Sometimes plans go astray and you will need to take emergency action:

- ○ Running out of time – jot down, in note form, the points that would have completed your essay. The examiner may give you some credit for this information.

- ○ Forgetting a name – do not waste time desperately trying to think of the name of a source. Indicate you know that the information is from another source by using a general reference like 'researchers have found'.

- ○ Forgetting facts or figures – if you have forgotten a piece of information, indicate to the examiner how you would go about finding it out. For example, if you have forgotten the side effects of a drug, describe how you would find them out.

## Action Points

1. Familiarise yourself with exam papers from previous years.

2. Make up mind maps for key topic areas.

3. Work with a friend on analysing a title and drawing up an essay plan. Set yourself a time limit and write an answer based on your plan.

---

## Summary Points

- ○ Summative assessments are set at the end of a study unit, term or academic year.

- ○ Preparation is the key to achieving a good standard of written work under exam conditions.

- ○ Find out how and when you will be assessed.

- Revise notes at consistent and regular intervals.
- Use mind maps to help in recall of information.
- Practise analysing the title, drafting a plan and writing an answer within a set time period.
- In the exam:
    - Read the paper carefully.
    - Choose questions wisely.
    - Make a plan.
- Leave time at the end to review your answer.

# 12

# Dissertations

A dissertation is an extended piece of written work that forms part of the final assessment on diploma courses and such like. It is distinguished from other essays submitted as coursework by its length and detailed treatment of its subject. Each student will make their own choice of topic, unlike set essays where all the students answer the same question. The content of the dissertation will represent the student's independent study of the subject matter, and will extend beyond the theory and practical applications formerly taught on the course.

Writing a dissertation provides the student with an opportunity to:

- study in depth one particular aspect of a subject
- learn the process of academic enquiry
- develop his or her thinking about a specific subject
- deal with a large amount of information
- be able to express ideas coherently
- sustain a discourse throughout a lengthy composition.

**Choosing a title**

Unlike set essays, where the question is chosen by the examiner, the student decides on the title for his or her dissertation. Although this is often the most challenging part of the task, it is important to get it right as it will shape both the structure and content of the essay. When writing your title the first step is to identify your topic.

### Deciding on the topic

You might already know your subject area. For instance, some courses contain advanced study units that involve the completion of a dissertation – so if you are studying ethics, your dissertation will be about some aspect of this. If you have more scope in choosing your topic, you may find Chapter 14 'Developing an Idea' useful.

A key point to consider is how interested you are in the topic. You will have to spend an enormous amount of time and effort in preparing your dissertation. By the completion of your project you may be less than enthusiastic about the work, so start with something that really excites you or has some personal significance for you. This will give you the impetus to keep going until the end.

Think about the feasibility of your project. Are the resources you need available? This will range from access to the appropriate journals and texts to a tutor who can offer you the appropriate supervision in developing your work.

### Refining the topic

Once you have a general idea of your subject matter, you can start to work at determining the focus of your enquiry. Use a brainstorm (see Chapter 5 'Letters and Reports') or a mind map (see Chapter 11 'Assessment') to generate ideas about different aspects of the topic. For example a brainstorm of 'cross-infection' might produce the keywords *Staphylococcus aureus*, antibiotics, wound infections, treatment, infection control measures and methicillin resistant *Staphylococcus aureus* (MRSA).

Once you have narrowed your search to a few keywords, you can start to think about the perspective you will take. Use question stems (Polit and Hungler 1995) to help define your enquiry. For example:

- o 'What is the cause of…?'

- o 'What are the consequences of…?'

- o 'How might…influence clinical practice?'

- o 'Is…still relevant?'

Dissertations are not about simply regurgitating all the facts you know about a particular topic. Look for causes, relationships and applications. Barnes (1995) suggests making a proposition and then questioning this. For example; 'Infection control measures have reduced the incidence of MRSA.' Do you agree? Is it possible to make this link? Questioning the proposition in this way prompts you to start examining relationships. In this case the association between the measures for controlling cross-infection and the incidence of MRSA is under scrutiny. Compare this with a more descriptive account of 'What is cross-infection?' Or 'What is the incidence of MRSA?'

Check that your choice of idea will produce enough material for you to be able to fulfil the requirements about length. There is no point starting on a topic that will produce only 3000 words when you are required to write 10,000. If you are sure that it will be sufficient you can start thinking about how you will phrase your title.

## Writing the title

You might want to write your title as a question or a statement. Whichever one you choose it must reflect the content of the dissertation and indicate your approach to the topic. Compare 'The role of infection control measures in reducing the incidence of MRSA' with 'A discussion about the limitations of current infection control measures in reducing the incidence of MRSA'. The approach taken by the writer is much clearer in the second title. Remember to keep the wording precise by eliminating any redundant words or phrases.

## The structure of your dissertation

Your dissertation is most likely to be analytical in nature. Use it to demonstrate your in-depth understanding of the subject matter and your ability to analyse and evaluate the information. The structure of your essay will be based on the keywords used in your title. These explain to the reader both your aims and your themes. What do you want to achieve with your work (for example, 'to explore x', 'to evaluate y' or 'to analyse z')? It is also important to identify the themes within your essay.

For example:

> A discussion about the limitations of current infection control measures in reducing the incidence of MRSA.

The key words are 'discussion', 'limitations', 'current infection control measures', 'reducing the incidence' and 'MRSA'.

The aims are 'to discuss' or 'to evaluate'.

The themes are:

- infection control measures
- MRSA (incidence of)
- the relationship between infection control and the incidence of MRSA.

The essay will examine the evidence for the effectiveness of infection control in reducing MRSA. This will involve evaluating the pros and the cons.

Breaking the essay down into its component parts in this way will help you organise information into a logical sequence. See Chapter 10 'Essays' for examples of different essay structures.

The use of headings is probably advisable considering the length of a dissertation. These might be usefully linked to the themes. For example, a section from the above essay might be headed 'The incidence of methicillin resistant *Staphyloccus aureus*'.

## Use your supervisor

Meet with your supervisor on a regular basis. He or she will be able to support your studies and advise on the writing up of your project. A good supervisor is an invaluable resource.

## References

A dissertation is a reflection of the broad and in-depth reading you have undertaken during your enquiry. It is vital that you acknowledge your sources by providing references. They will help distinguish your original thoughts and ideas from those of other researchers. The nature of these references will also give an indication of whether the information you have used is current or not and the validity of your source material. Supplying a complete and comprehensive reference list will enable the reader to follow up sources for themselves.

There are two main styles of referencing:

- the Harvard style
- the Vancouver style.

### The Harvard style

The Harvard or 'author–date' system is well known and widely used within academic institutions.

For books, the name of the author and the year of publication are placed in parentheses within the main body of the text, for example:

Use question stems (Polit and Hungler 1995) to help define your enquiry.'

Use the date of publication that accompanies the copyright sign on the title page. Do not use the date of reprints. However, if there is more than one edition of the book then use the date of the revision or edition you are using.

Include a reference to figures or tables along with author name and date if you are directly referring to this.

Direct quotes or references to specific parts of a text must be accompanied by the author, date and inclusive page numbers.

If your reference is part of the text then no parentheses are used for the names. For example, 'Barnes (1995) suggests…'

Initials are not provided in the text unless you are quoting two different authors with the same last name.

References to works by the same author and published within the same year can be distinguished by adding a suffix letter, for example Argyle 1983a.

List single author publications first, before co-authored works where the single author is the first name to appear, for example:

Argyle 1983

Argyle and McHenry 1971.

Several references by the same author or authors should be listed chronologically.

Where two or more references are made to different authors to support a single point, then list authors and separate them with a semicolon, for example: (Flesch 1948; Gunning 1952).

Full references are provided in an alphabetical list at the end of the work. This list will contain all references contained within the main body of the text, for example:

Polit, D. and Hungler, B. (1995) *Essentials of Nursing Research: Methods, Appraisal and Utilization (5th edition). Philadelphia, PA: Lippincott.*

Note the order of the information.

For books:

- o author's last name
- o initials
- o date of publication
- o title
- o edition if applicable
- o place of publication
- o Publisher.

For edited books:

- o editor's last name
- o initials
- o date of publication
- o title
- o edition if applicable
- o place of publication
- o publisher.

Articles in journals have the following order:

- o author's last name
- o initials
- o date of publication
- o title of article
- o title of journal
- o volume and part number of journal
- o pages (inclusive).

For example:

> Ong, G., Austoker, J. and Brouwer, A. (1996) 'Evaluation of the Written Information Sent to Women who are Called Back for Further Investigation of Breast Screening in the UK.' *Health Education Journal 55*, 4, 413–429.

For articles in books:

- ○ author's last name
- ○ initials
- ○ date of publication
- ○ title of article
- ○ 'In:'
- ○ names of editors
- ○ title of book
- ○ place of publication
- ○ publisher.

For official reports:

- ○ name of the government department
- ○ date of publication
- ○ title of report
- ○ reference number
- ○ place of publication
- ○ publisher.

For theses:

- ○ author's last name
- ○ initials
- ○ date of publication
- ○ title of thesis
- ○ type of thesis (MSc, PhD)
- ○ Name of academic institution where thesis was submitted.

For papers from the proceedings of a conference:

- ○ last name of author
- ○ initials
- ○ names of editors
- ○ year of publication
- ○ title of paper

- ○  'In:'
- ○  title of conference proceedings
- ○  place of conference
- ○  date of conference
- ○  inclusive page numbers
- ○  place of publication
- ○  publisher.

For an unpublished conference paper:

- ○  last name of author
- ○  initials
- ○  year paper presented
- ○  title of paper
- ○  'Presented at:'
- ○  title of conference
- ○  place of conference
- ○  date of conference
- ○  inclusive page numbers
- ○  'Unpublished'.

For a newspaper article (unsigned):

- ○  name of newspaper
- ○  date of publication
- ○  title of article
- ○  page numbers.

For a personal communication (information given to you informally, for example by phone or by letter):

- ○  last name of the communicator
- ○  initials
- ○  date on which communication took place, followed by
- ○  'Personal Communication'.

Note that only the first letter of the title and proper nouns are given in capitals. Information in the reference list is always given in full; however, some references may be abbreviated in the text:

- two authors – both names are used

- more than two authors – give the name of the first author plus 'et al.'

A standard form of abbreviation for journal titles may be acceptable if they have been approved internationally.

### The Vancouver style

The Vancouver style is often favoured in nursing publications. Numbers instead of the names of authors are used within the text. These numbers correspond with the reference list provided at the end of the book or article. This list is organised according to the assigned number instead of being arranged alphabetically, for example:

'Use question stems (3)' or 'Use question stems'[3]

Note that the numbers appear either in brackets or in an elevated position.

References to more than one source would use inclusive numbers, for example 2–5.

References to any figure or table must be given if you are directly referring to this, for example (3 Figure 4.5).

In the reference list it would appear as:

3. Polit, D. and Hungler, B. *Essentials of Nursing Research:
Methods, Appraisal and Utilization (5th edition). Philadelphia, PA:
Lippincott, 1995.*

Note that the type and order of information in the reference list is the same as the Harvard style except that the date of publication is placed at the end of the journal title or at the end of the whole entry for books.

Referencing styles vary between academic institutions, journals and publishing houses. Always check out the guidelines before you start compiling your reference list. Entering the details using the recommended format right at the start of your project will save you a lot of editing time later.

Regardless of which style of referencing you use there must be sufficient information in the text to enable the reader to track the source in the reference list. This list should contain information about all of the material (both written and unwritten) used by the writer to prepare the composition. It will correspond exactly with the references cited in the main body of the text.

Sometimes a bibliography is given in addition to the reference list. It will contain details of material that has influenced the writer during the preparation of their work. There are no direct references to this material in the main body of the text. Sometimes bibliographies are used to suggest further reading.

### Submission

Ask your tutor or refer to your institutional guidelines about the presentation and submission of your essay. It is vital that you comply with these otherwise you may lose marks or have your essay rejected.

See Chapter 10 'Essays' for some general advice on preparing essays for submission. The final word – remember the effort and time you have put into preparing your dissertation needs to be rewarded with a good quality binder that does not fall apart in the marker's hands.

---

## Summary Points

- A dissertation is an extended piece of written work that forms part of the final assessment on diploma courses and such like.

- Writing a dissertation is an opportunity for you to study in depth one particular aspect of a subject and learn about the process of academic enquiry.

- Use a brainstorm or a mind map to generate ideas about topics.

- Dissertations are analytical in nature and are about causes, relationships and applications.

- The structure of a dissertation will be based on the keywords used in the title. These keywords explain to the reader both the aims and the themes of the essay.

- Sources must always be acknowledged. There are two styles of referencing – the Harvard and the Vancouver.

- Always comply with your institution's guidelines about presentation and submission.

# 13

# Research Projects

The final year assessment on many health courses involves the presentation of a thesis based on original research carried out by the student. This research paper will describe in detail the investigation planned and carried out by the student.

Writing up these research projects helps the student to:

○ develop critical appraisal skills as he or she reviews the literature

○ understand the scientific language used to describe the research process

○ learn about the mechanics and style of academic writing

○ learn to evaluate the strengths and weaknesses of his or her own work

○ receive validation of his or her work via the assessment system.

The following chapter offers the student who is about to embark on his or her first research paper advice on how to organise and structure such research reports.

## The structure of your research paper

All researchers must know how to present their investigations and findings in written form. Fortunately such papers have a traditional structure that makes it easier for the novice to organise his or her material into a coherent and scientific account. You will find that this well-established pattern mirrors the research process. The report will tell the reader the why (your reason for carrying out the research), the how (your methods of investigation) and the what (what are your findings?).

The contents of a research paper will be divided into the following sections:

- summary
- introduction
- literature review
- methods
- results
- discussion
- conclusion.

Compare this with the research process:

- Why? – the question or problem is discussed in the 'introduction' and 'literature review'.
- How? – how you studied the problem or investigated the question is described in the section on 'methods'.
- What? – your findings will be detailed in the section on 'results' and an evaluation provided under the 'discussion'.

A summary of this research process is usually placed at the beginning of the research thesis.

**If your research is *quantitative* use the following guidelines.**

### *In your summary*
Most papers start with a summary of the main points of the research. It provides the reader with an outline of the study using about 250 words. Briefly state your objectives, design and methods along with your findings and conclusions.

### *In your introduction*
State the research hypotheses you are investigating. Give brief details of any relevant background information.

Write why you think your research will be useful or pertinent. For example, does it have a practical application? How does it contribute to the evidence base of the profession?

### In your literature review

Use this section to review other studies relevant to your project. This will help set your work within the context of the current state of research in your chosen area. The reader will gain an idea of the questions or problems that other researchers are studying and the results of these investigations. Make the links between your research and the other studies clear. How are you building on this evidence base? How will your project extend scientific knowledge?

A literature review is not just about regurgitating sequentially the facts and figures of various studies. You must show the examiner that you are able to draw information together and summarise the findings of studies that are in agreement, for instance ones that have similar findings or those using the same methodology.

Show the examiner that you are able to critically appraise the evidence. Why is the study relevant to your research? Do you agree with the evaluation of the findings? Is the design valid? Were the methods of data collection reliable? What is the significance of their contribution to scientific knowledge or clinical practice? Remember to take a broad perspective that encompasses both those studies that are in accordance and those that oppose each other.

Use the final part of this section to give more details of your planned research. You will need to:

○   state your aims or objectives

○   restate your hypotheses

○   state the dependent and independent variables

○   state your rationale for designing the research

○   state the scope and depth of the project

○   state definitions of terminology where appropriate.

### In your methods section

The methods section tells the reader how you went about answering your question or investigating the problem. It must contain enough detail to ensure that another researcher is able to replicate your project. This information will also help the reader to appraise the strengths and weaknesses of your research.

Divide the information into subsections that cover the:

- design
- subjects
- materials or equipment
- procedure.

*Your design*

State your design (for example, repeated measures, matched subjects) and your rationale for making this choice.

Discuss any pilot studies you have carried out and how this has affected your choice of design.

Describe how your subjects were allocated to the experimental and control groups.

State your independent and dependent variables.

*The subjects*

Describe your sample (for example, size, type). State the criteria you used to select your subjects.

*Materials or equipment*

Be specific about your materials or apparatus (for example, any technical equipment you used or the content of a questionnaire). Include diagrams where appropriate.

*The procedure*

Describe exactly what was done (for example, how did you control for situational variables?)

Describe what each subject experienced during the procedure (for example, the instructions received from the researcher).

Describe how the data was collected.

Describe how the data was analysed.

State the statistical test and level of probability used in the experiment.

Give your rationale for your choice of data collection and analysis.

*Ethical issues*

Describe any ethical issues that arose out of your study and how you dealt with them. Include information about obtaining permission from the relevant ethics committee. It would also be useful to briefly note how you have ensured client confidentiality.

### In your results

This section contains the results of your enquiry. What have you found out? Provide a summary of the data within the text and place the full version in the appendices. Visual displays like tables and graphs are invaluable for presenting numerical information. See below on how to use these displays effectively.

Remember there is no interpretation of the data in this section as this is reserved for the discussion section that follows.

### In your discussion

This section is about making sense of and interpreting the significance of your findings. It is useful to start this section by restating your aims. This helps focus the reader and reminds him or her of your original objectives as stated in the literature review.

Write your interpretation of your results. Are your hypotheses rejected or accepted? How do your results compare with the findings of the studies in your literature review? Where does your research fit into the overall picture? Have you attempted to explain any inconsistencies or unexpected findings? Are you able to put forward any alternative hypotheses?

Make an objective evaluation of the strengths and weaknesses of your project. Describe how you might modify or extend your research project in the light of this evaluation.

Describe what the implications of your project might be for developing theoretical knowledge or clinical practice.

### In your conclusion

Draw your report to a close by reiterating the main points.

Use your appendices for:

- ○ the full version of your raw data
- ○ copies of statistical calculations or computer analyses
- ○ examples of materials used in data collection, for example copies of scoring sheets, instructions or questionnaires.

**If your research is** *qualitative*, the structure of your research report will be very similar to the style used for quantitative research. However there are some major differences.

In your introduction and literature review:

- As yours is not an experimental design, you will not have hypotheses as such. However, you do need to state your research question or problem.

- You must give a greater emphasis to describing your theoretical and methodological framework.

In your methods:

- Your description of subjects and the context of your research will be in much greater depth.

- Explain how your planned investigation is appropriate for your objectives.

In your results and discussion:

- The results and discussion sections are usually combined.

- The results are more likely to be narrative – and relate to themes and categories – rather than numerical. This makes it more difficult to present them clearly to the reader. However, you must show enough data in the main part of your paper to demonstrate your findings.

- Although the two sections are combined you must clearly make the distinction between the data you have collected and your analysis.

- Show how you have selected and interpreted your data in your analysis.

- Like a researcher who carries out a quantitative research project, you will want to reflect on the research process itself. For example, how reliable were your observations and measurements?

- You will also want to reflect on your role as the researcher. This is a fundamental difference between quantitative and qualitative research. What preconceptions did you hold? What influence might you have made on data collection? Have you created a bias in the selection of subjects? For instance, a student researcher might select fellow students to take part in his or her study .

- Support your analysis by reference to other studies.

## References

It is essential that you indicate the source of material by providing clear references both within the text and in a reference list at the end of your paper. Make a clear distinction between your original ideas and those of other researchers. For instance, you need to provide a reference with a small amount of information if you are replicating another experiment.

Plagiarism is considered a serious matter by all institutions. You may lose a considerable amount of marks or be failed if it is considered that you are presenting another researcher's work as your own. See Chapter 12 'Dissertations' for information on how to present references. You will also need to check your institution's guidelines on the expected format of referencing.

## How to display numerical data

Use visual displays to present your numerical data. These will make it easier for your reader to understand your results, recognise trends and identify patterns within the data.

### Tables

Tables can show either a complete record of your original data or a summary of essential information. They are a useful way of presenting complex data especially when it is repetitive in nature. Tables help to organise information and illustrate patterns for the reader. For example, a table might be used to provide a summary of information about your research subjects.

Design tips:

◊  Always indicate your units of measurement.

◊  Choose symbols or icons for use in tables carefully. Do they already have a universal meaning? For instance, a tick is usually seen as positive.

◊  Figures listed in columns are easier to read than numbers presented in rows.

◊  Place sets of data to be compared next to each other on the page.

### Graphs

Graphs are a simple but effective way to represent your data. Your choice of display will depend on the level of measurement used in your experiment. This will be at either a nominal, ordinal or interval level.

*Nominal level data* – subjects or items are classified into categories. For example, subjects may be assigned to categories according to discipline (dental, physiotherapy, nursing) or location (hospital A, hospital B).

*Ordinal level data* – scores are assigned to subjects or items according to a particular characteristic. These scores are then used to rank the subjects or items from the highest to the lowest. Rating is done using subjective measures so that the size of the interval between points is not guaranteed to be identical. For example, students might be ranked on levels of motivation using a ten point scale with ten as the highest. A student scoring nine is relatively higher in motivation than one scoring two. However, the interval between points one and two is not known to be exactly the same as that between points eight and nine.

*Interval level data* – scores are ranged on a scale where the intervals between points are equal. Examples of measurements on an interval scale are time, weight, temperature, age and blood pressure.

For *nominal* level data use:

- bar charts
- pie charts.

### Bar charts

There are different types of bar chart that include vertical, horizontal, multiple and proportional.

#### Vertical bar charts

Each category is represented by a vertical bar, the height of which relates to the numerical value of that category. Use vertical bar charts to show comparisons between categories. Figure 13.1 compares the waiting times for day surgery at three different hospitals.

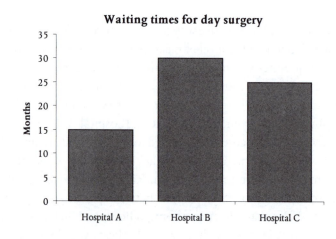

*Figure 13.1  A vertical bar chart*

Design tips:

◊   Indent the first bar so that it is set away from the y axis.

### Horizontal bar charts

Each category is represented by a horizontal bar, the length of which represents the numerical value of the data. This type of bar chart shows comparisons between categories at a single point in time. Figure 13.2 allows us to compare the number of failed appointments in three different disciplines during one month.

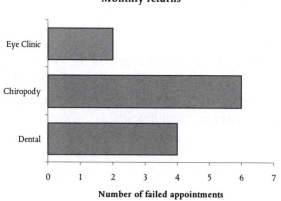

*Figure 13.2 A horizontal bar chart*

Design tip:

◊ Write the names of the categories instead of having a y axis.

### Multiple bar charts

Multiple bar charts show comparisons between related sets of categories. In Figure 13.3 the side effects of three different drugs are compared.

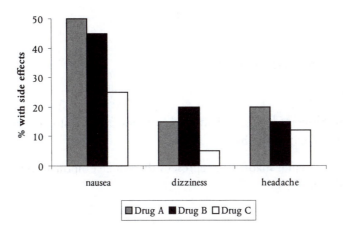

**Comparison of side effects**

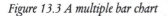

*Figure 13.3 A multiple bar chart*

Design tips:

◊ Use different kinds of shading to provide a contrast between each bar.

◊ Use the same kind of shading for each category, so they are instantly recognisable.

### Proportional bar charts

These charts are also known as stratified, stacked or component bar charts. They show the division of the whole into its relative proportions. Each bar represents the whole, and each segment part of that whole. It is possible to make comparisons between both the whole and the constituent parts. Figure 13.4 shows the number of beds in different specialities across three hospitals.

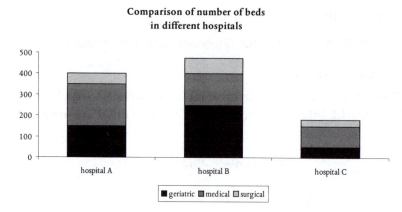

*Figure 13.4 A proportional bar chart*

Design tips:

◊ Use different kinds of shading to provide a contrast between each component of the bar.

◊ Use the same shading to represent the same component on different bars.

*Pie charts*

Pie charts are useful for giving a general impression of the data; however, they give less information than other types of visual display. Use them to show what proportions make up a whole, rather than specific details of figures. The pie chart in Figure 13.5 illustrates the types of referral to an occupational therapy service.

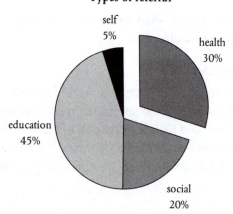

*Figure 13.5 A pie chart*

Design tips:

◊ Limit categories to a maximum of six.

◊ Start segments at the 12 o'clock position.

  ○ Use different kinds of shading for the segments.

  ○ Explode out segments you want to highlight.

  ○ Avoid comparisons between two or more pie charts, as this tends to be less effective.

For grouped data of at least *ordinal* level use:

  ○ histograms

  ○ frequency polygons.

*Histograms*

A histogram shows the frequency distribution of scores. The x axis is marked off in units that can represent either single scores (1, 2, 3) or scores arranged into groups (1–5, 6–10). The height of the bar on the y axis represents the frequency of the individual score or group of scores. Figure 13.6 shows the data from an experiment about the effects of sleep deprivation on the scores of a verbal reasoning test. It is clear that the control scores are higher than the experimental scores.

*Effects of Sleep Deprivation*

## 1. Experimental group

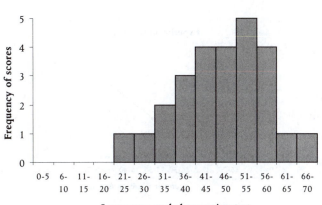

*Figure 13.6a A histogram*

**2. Control Group**

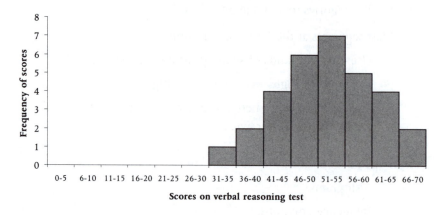

*Figure 13.6b A histogram*

Design tips:

◊   There are no gaps between the bars.

*Frequency polygons*

The bars of the histogram are replaced by points plotted at the midpoint of the top of each bar. When these points are joined up you have a frequency polygon (see Figure 13.7). The height of the dots on the y axis represents the frequency of the score. Choose a polygon rather than a histogram if you want to display two or more sets of data on one graph.

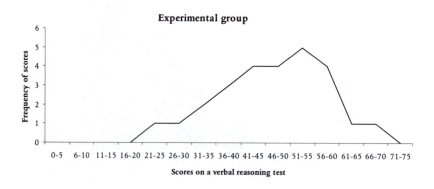

*Figure 13.7 A frequency polygon*

Design tips:

◊ Bring the ends of the polygon down to zero.

For data values on a continuous scale of at least *ordinal* level use:

- ○ line graphs
- ○ scattergrams.

*Line graphs*

Use line graphs for data at ordinal or interval level. They are useful for showing either consistency or changes over time. Figure 13.8 compares the weight loss of three different clients.

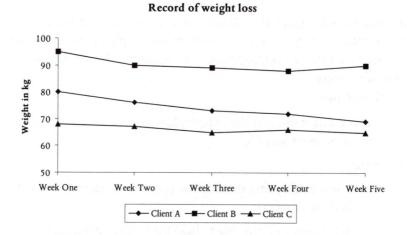

*13.8 A line graph*

Design tips:

◊ Avoid overcomplicating the graph by trying to display too many lines at a time.

◊ Try to differentiate between lines in some way, for example a bold versus a dotted line.

◊ Use bold to emphasise the most important line where appropriate.

*Scattergrams*

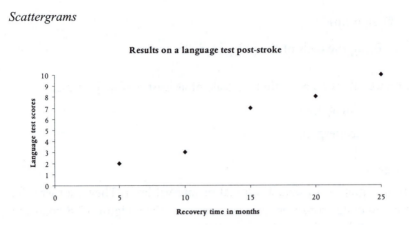

*Figure 13.9 A scattergram*

A scattergram is a graph that allows you to use a dot to represent an individual result. In Figure 13.9 each point on the graph represents the score of a stroke client on a language test (y axis) compared with the length of time of recovery.

Design tips:

◊ The x axis is used for the independent variable and the y axis for the dependent variable.

In general:

○ Use a display that shows what your results mean rather than just the numbers.

○ Use labels and captions to help the reader interpret the material.

○ Draw graphs carefully so that the accuracy of the data is not affected by poor execution.

○ Break down a complex graph into two or three simpler ones.

○ Always display time on the horizontal axis.

○ Visual displays need to be:

   ○ accurate

   ○ clear

   ○ comprehensible

○   unambiguous

○   appropriate for the data.

## Submitting your project

Ask your tutor or refer to your institutional guidelines about presentation and submission of your research project. It is vital that you comply with these otherwise you may lose marks or have your project rejected.

In general, research projects must be:

○   Typed – all institutions require research projects to be either typed or word-processed on one side of good quality A4 paper.

○   Bound – research projects must be bound in the special folders available from your institution. Completed projects are kept in the library and are available for reference to other students.

○   Well spaced – make sure you have adequate margins. The left-hand margin needs to be wider to allow for binding.

○   Easy to read – keep lines well spaced and use a font size of at least 12 points.

○   Paginated – check guidelines on how pages should be numbered. Roman numerals are sometimes used for the list of contents, list of figures and acknowledgements. The main part of the project should be in Arabic numerals.

○   In order – most institutions will require projects to be presented in the following way.

  ○   Front sheet with:

  ○   the project title

  ○   your name

  ○   your tutor's name

  ○   the title of your course

  ○   the year of submission.

(Start each one of the following on a separate sheet.)

- ○ List of contents
- ○ List of tables (include the reference number, title and page number)
- ○ List of figures (include the reference number, title and page number)
- ○ List of appendices (include the reference number or letter, title and page number)
- ○ Acknowledgements (include name of supervisor and other key advisors or supporters)
- ○ Summary
- ○ Introduction
- ○ Literature review
- ○ Methodology
- ○ Results
- ○ Discussion
- ○ Appendices
- ○ Reference list
- ○ Bibliography.

## Action Points

1. Study the theses of former students. Look at how they have structured their paper. What information did they include under the different sections? Is any information missing? Is it clear?

## Summary Points

- Students are often required as part of their final assessment to present a thesis based on their own original research.

- Writing such reports helps the student to develop critical appraisal skills, understand scientific language and write in the style appropriate for an academic composition.

- The structure of these reports mirrors the research process itself. They are usually divided into the following sections:

  - Summary

  - Introduction

  - Literature review

  - Methods

  - Results

  - Discussion.

- An important part of writing the report is the student's ability to make an objective evaluation of the strengths and weaknesses of his or her project.

- In qualitative research this is extended to the ability of the student to reflect on his or her role as the researcher.

- Acknowledgement of other sources is essential. There must be a clear distinction between the student's original ideas and the work of other researchers.

## PART THREE

# Writing for Publication

# Writing for Publication

There are many opportunities for health professionals to write and be published. They range from whole books to chapters, journal articles or features in newspapers and magazines. There are various academic levels, styles and approaches to suit the needs of every writer.

Writing and being published is both a personal and professional achievement. Publication provides a forum for disseminating information, sharing ideas and initiating debate amongst health professionals.

The main section of this part of the book looks at different aspects of writing, starting with developing an idea and planning a schedule through to writing styles and ways of presenting a manuscript.

The final section offers advice on three specific types of writing – journal articles, books and media pieces.

## Developing an Idea

Finding out what is on the market. Brainstorming ideas. Testing out your idea.

## Managing Your Time Effectively

Planning your schedule. Setting up a timetable. Tips for making better use of your time.

## Determining Your Style

Structuring a piece of writing. Checking for ambiguities, confusions and errors.

### Getting the Best Out of Your Personal Computer

Organising and storing your work. Working with a co-author. Checklist for authors buying a computer.

### Presenting Your Work

Hints on page layout. Styles of text. Spelling. Organising your manuscript for submission.

### Protecting Your Rights

Contracts. Copyright.

## Publication Skills in Context

### Journal Articles

Finding the right journal. Structuring your article. The role of reviewers.

### Books

Single author or collaborative writing. Writing and submitting a proposal. Ten tips to beat writer's block.

### Articles for the Media

Aspects of writing for the media. Finding a market. Writing a query letter. Writing your article.

# 14

# Writing for Publication
## Developing an Idea

You may be lucky enough to already have some ideas about what to write. However, it is more likely that you have decided to write but you are stuck for an idea. Try stimulating your imagination through the following.

## Browsing

Find out the topics health professionals are currently writing about by browsing through recently published material. Check out publications in a range of disciplines and not just your own. This will help you have a greater understanding of both the issues and the approaches to writing that are currently popular.

Looking at other authors' work can also help provide some inspiration. Comparing approaches by different authors to the same subject can lift away some of the unconscious boundaries that restrict creativity. For example, anatomy may seem a very dry subject, but one author saw the potential for a colour by numbers book for students. Another author combined two different styles within the same book, so the reader was able to choose between using it as an A to Z directory or to follow a theme using trails marked by the author.

### Browsing through books

Check the description of new titles in catalogues, bookstores, libraries or on the World Wide Web. Are there any ideas that you might adapt to suit your area of expertise? Can you contribute information or advice that would be of use to other disciplines?

### Browsing through professional articles

Most hospitals and community services provide staff libraries that subscribe to a wide range of health and health-related journals. Skim articles or at least read their abstracts. Look at a range of articles, and not just those written specifically for your discipline. What are the current topics of interest? Who are the authors? What are the common approaches?

### Browsing through the media

Copies of the main newspapers and some magazines are available at your local library. Alternatively borrow from friends or read through a selection in the waiting room of your local dentist or GP. Study the topics that are currently in vogue. What type of article is of interest to the general public?

## Reflecting

Use your own clinical experience to identify who and what you want to write about.

Ask yourself:

- What questions are most frequently asked by my clients?
- What are their common concerns or misunderstandings?
- Are the materials available that I would like to give to my clients?

(The answers may lead to ideas about books and articles written specifically for clients.)

- What written materials for other disciplines would help support my work?
- Is there a gap in practical resource books for use for work with clients?
- Have I developed written materials to help in educating clients?

(The answers may lead to ideas about practical resource books or advice articles for use by colleagues or other disciplines.)

- Am I using an innovative treatment approach?
- Do I have an example of best practice to share?
- Have I completed a piece of research?

(The answers may lead to books and articles for use by colleagues or other disciplines.)

- Do I want to share my experience in training others?
- Do I feel there is a need for written materials to support students?
- Do I have extensive or specialist knowledge of a particular area?

(The answers may lead to introductory or advanced textbooks, training manuals or continuing education articles.)

## Brainstorming

Brainstorming is a useful technique if you know your topic but need to be more specific. For example, the subject of asthma is a common and very topical subject. However, it may be approached in many different ways depending on the author and the market. The following examples all concern asthma, but each one differs in perspective and its target readership:

- an article in a monthly parents' magazine by a reader giving a personal account of living with a child with asthma
- a newspaper story about new traffic measures to reduce car pollution in an area with a high incidence of childhood asthma
- a journal article describing a research project investigating the effect of motivational interviewing on changing the lifestyle habits of chronic asthma sufferers
- a guide for parents on helping their adolescent child cope with asthma
- an article by a school nurse in a journal for teachers giving information about managing the child with asthma in school
- a textbook for medical students on the diagnosis, treatment and management of asthma.

## Reviewing

Have you ever found yourself making any of the following comments on something you have read?

- ○ 'It's okay as far as it goes...'
- ○ 'What I really wanted was...'
- ○ 'Parents really need to know this but the language is far too complicated...'
- ○ 'This book is too advanced for my students...'

Critically reviewing other publications is one way to identify gaps or opportunities.

### Enquiring

Talk to the publishers. Find out from the commissioning editors the topics they are currently seeking.

### Test out your idea

Eureka! You have an idea, but before you go any further you need to know if your idea is a sound one.

◊ Will it sink or swim?

Make sure that you have got the necessary knowledge and skills to complete the project. The majority of writers will need to do some research to help develop and expand their original concept, so there is no need for you to have all the answers at the beginning. However, no matter how great your idea, you must be completely confident that you can see it through. If not, your idea will sink without trace.

◊ Is there enough substance to it?

Your initial idea must have the potential to be developed into a piece of writing that will engage the readers' interest and be informative. Be flexible with ideas. You may not have enough for a book, but it might well suit an article.

◊ Is it original?

It is all too easy to think you have come up with a wonderful new concept. You may then be surprised how many other people have had the very same thought. Always do your market research carefully. This way you will be aware if somebody has already 'written your article or book'.

◊  Is it marketable?

You may be very enthusiastic about this particular subject and be
happy to spend long hours reading and studying about it. However,
unless the potential readers feel the same, you are unlikely to get it accepted for publication. Be realistic about how many people will want
to read your choice of subject matter.

◊  Why you?

It is often fruitful to think about why you should be writing the article and not somebody else. What can you offer? This can help you refine your basic idea so that it is unique to you.

Has your idea passed the test? Yes? Then you are ready to proceed. Check
out chapters 20 to 22 on writing books, journal articles or media articles.

**Action Points**

1.   Make an 'ideas' file.

Professional writers often collect reference material that is related to their
field of interest. If you intend to commit yourself to writing on a regular
basis, then I would definitely recommend that you start accumulating data
in this way.

As with any other compilation, you will need some sort of filing system, otherwise you will spend hours trying to retrieve the information you
require. File material alphabetically or in subject groups using a concertina
file, filing cabinet or box files. Regularly updating an index will mean you
can access material quickly.

Items that might be included are journal articles, newspaper cuttings,
magazine interviews, book reviews and even cartoons. Keep a section on
'sound bites'. These might include quotes from public speakers, a presenter's comments on television or even a joke you heard from a friend.

The file will provide a source of inspiration as well as a ready supply of
reference material. Browse through your collection whenever you need
help to generate some ideas.

## Summary Points

○ Browse through recently published material to find out the current topics written by health professionals.

○ Use your own clinical experience to identify who and what you want to write about.

○ Brainstorm different approaches to the same topic.

○ Critically review other publications to identify gaps or opportunities for offering a different approach or perspective.

○ Find out what topics the publishers are currently seeking.

○ Make sure you have the skills and knowledge to complete the task.

○ Choose an idea that is original with an easily identified target readership.

# 15

# Managing Your Time Effectively

Writing, whether it is part of study, research or for publication, is time-consuming. It requires careful planning to ensure that you produce a quality piece of work, as well as being able to meet your deadlines. Early preparation will help you identify your priorities and create a realistic work schedule. Regular monitoring of the way that you are using your time will keep you focused and on task. You will also be more able to cope with unforeseen circumstances or changes to your initial goals.

This chapter offers advice about applying time-management techniques to your writing project. These strategies are usually associated with business, and you may question their relevance for something as aesthetic as writing. However, it should help you do *what* you want to do, *when* you want to do it – helping creativity, rather than hindering it.

## Planning your schedule

You may have already started setting up a timetable in which you have selected certain days and times for 'writing'. Regular slots are important in establishing the writing habit, but you still need to plan how to use this time in the most effective way. This will involve the same processes and strategies required in the formulation of any project. You will need to set goals, identify the resource implications and consider the timeframe needed to complete your writing.

### *Setting your goals*

Your first step in planning your writing is to be very clear about your final objective. Be as precise as possible. Think about exactly what you want to achieve, and the date by which you want it completed. Write this down in a statement. For example, 'write 1500 word article on "The Role of the

Health Visitor in Managing Feeding Difficulties in the Pre-School Child"
for publication in the November edition of *Health Visiting Today*'.

Your next step is to start planning the work required to meet your objective. Think of your project in terms of clearly defined stages. Start by
identifying the sequence of steps that are common to all writing tasks.
These will include researching and planning your work, plus the main task
of actually writing and probably rewriting it several times, as well as the final stages required in preparing your manuscript for the publishers. Do not
forget to include those post-submission tasks like reading proofs.

Once you have some idea of the overall sequence of events you can
start to identify the main goals related to each stage. (For larger projects it
may help to divide each stage into smaller units that relate either to chapter
headings, sections or specific theoretical areas.) In the above example, one
of your main goals might be to research 'feeding difficulties'.

Now you need to list the tasks you need to perform in order to reach
your goals. For the above goal your tasks might include:

  ○  browsing books, articles and other information sources

  ○  identifying seminal texts

  ○  reading recent research

  ○  reviewing notes from conferences/courses

  ○  making notes.

Make a list of the things you need to do in order to fulfil each task. Be as
specific and concrete as possible. For instance, you might decide to carry
out a database search to help in reading current research on feeding difficulties. Ask yourself questions to help refine the task. What do you consider as current? This will help you in specifying the time interval for your
search. Are you interested in findings only in the United Kingdom or
worldwide? Again this will help in setting some parameters around your
search. Which feeding difficulties interest you? This will help you in carrying out your search and in selecting the appropriate databases.

When you have answered these questions you should have a more precise description of the task. This is easily translated into a mini-target. The
above example could be phrased as 'to complete a search on European research into refusal of food by infants between two and five years of age, using CINAHL, ClinPSYC and PsychLit from 1990 to current time'. Precise
targets are easier to measure, and therefore more useful in indicating
whether or not you have achieved your goals.

At first it will be difficult to break down your project into a very detailed analysis. However, you need to have a clear idea of your overall goals before you can start thinking about the timeframe, so aim to identify as much detail as possible. Use the planning sheet in Figure 15.1 to start filling in your main goals and subgoals. You can expand on your original plan as you work on your project. It may be helpful to make a few copies of the planner so that you can redraft your plan as needed.

Review your list of goals and start to prioritise. Although there will be a natural sequence, some things will need to be done very early on. For example, obtaining copyright to reproduce a table or diagram can take some time. If you can identify this at the outset, you can apply for permission in plenty of time.

In summary, you need to:

- Write a clear and specific statement about your final objective.
- Determine the sequence of stages needed to meet this objective.
- Identify the main goals required to complete each stage.
- List the tasks you need to perform in order to fulfil these goals.
- Ask yourself questions to help refine each task and identify mini-targets.
- Review and prioritise as necessary.

### Resources

All good planning involves some forethought about the resources needed to complete a project. The following factors need to be considered:

- space
- equipment
- helpers
- information.

Space – you will need at least an area you can call your own that includes a space for writing. Is this already available or will you need time to set this up? For instance, do you have to clear all your junk out of the spare room before you can make it into your study!

## Planning Sheet

subgoals

Goal _____ By:

1 _____

2 _____

3 _____

Goal _____ By:

1 _____

2 _____

3 _____

Goal _____ By:

1 _____

2 _____

3 _____

Final completion date _____

*Figure 15.1*

Equipment – list all the equipment you think you will need for the project. Remember to include minor items, like paper and files, to major investments like desks, shelves and even computers. Do you need to order items? You may have to wait, which again will impact on your timescale.

Helpers – you are not likely to be employing a staff group. However, you do need to consider the needs of other people who may be assisting you. For instance, you will need to check the availability of typists, and ask for an estimate of how long they will need to do the job.

Information – this applies to information in libraries, databases, the Internet and so on. Remember to check access and opening times of libraries. Unfortunately access is becoming more and more restricted so it may take time and planning in applying for membership. Remember that university libraries restrict opening times over holiday periods. Check with staff that there are no planned closures. It is surprising how the most unlikely events occur just as you desperately need access to the library – major computer updating, strikes, refurbishment or relocation, to name but a few.

Each one of the above can impact on your timing, so they need to be considered in advance and your timetable adjusted accordingly.

### Timeframe

You should now have a clear plan with identified objectives, and an idea of the resources you require to meet those goals. Before finalising your timeframe, there are a few more factors to think about.

Available time – do you know how much time you have available to work on your project? Before you can manage your time more effectively, you need to know how you are using your time at the moment. Look at the 'Action Points' at the end of this chapter to find out more about how to complete and analyse an activity record. This will help reveal the patterns in your daily life. Are you using your time in the most effective and efficient way at the moment? If not, you may need to re-establish your priorities and organise your time accordingly.

External constraints – there is no point in having your heart set on a particular date if this is unsuitable for the publisher's schedule or if a journal needs to have your article six months ahead of publication. Check out all the possible constraints.

Personal goals – do you want your work published within a certain year or in a particular quarterly journal? This will give you a very firm target to work towards, but you must make sure that it is a realistic goal.

Writing style – you will need to estimate how long you personally need to complete the task. There are individual differences in writing style and ability. Think about how you work best. This might be in short, intensive bursts or at a slow, steady pace over a longer period of time. Be realistic. Set a timetable that reflects the speed and manner of your writing.

Workload – look at the goals on your planning schedule. Do you need to research background information, or do you have most of your data ready? When will you be ready to start writing up a draft? You may need to allow for a longer period of time for researching your material. How big is your project? A manuscript of 120,000 words requires a very different timescale to a smaller project of 60,000 words. Can you achieve this amount of work within the planned dates? Again, be realistic.

Co-authors – co-authors need to negotiate timeframes carefully. Problems can arise if different writing styles have not been addressed in the planning stage. The timetable should meet the needs of each individual, and this often means going with the lowest common denominator. There is no point one person racing ahead if the other author is still methodically but slowly working through his or her own work. Remember to include additional slots for meetings, sharing work, joint planning and editing sessions.

Other considerations – major events, whether personal, social or work, need to be taken into account. Allow for time out for such things as major business trips, family weddings or planned hospital treatment.

You are now ready to make an estimate of how much time you will need to complete each stage. Work backwards from your finish date and mark in completion dates for each stage on your plan. Remember that it is commonplace for articles for peer-reviewed journals to be returned for re-drafting, and editors may return your chapter or book with queries or corrections requiring your attention. These factors need to be taken into consideration when planning your schedule.

### Setting up a timetable

Use your planner to draw up a timetable that includes weekly or monthly schedules covering your intended timeframe. Block out time committed to non-writing activities like work, shopping, a hobby or family activities like taking the children swimming. Remember to include one-off events like weddings, holidays or work situations such as attending a major conference.

You should be left with blank squares that represent your writing time. Draw your timetable large enough so that there is space to write in daily goals.

Use your planning sheet to mark the completion dates for your subgoals, main goals and stages on the timetable. If you find that one of your completion dates coincides with a major event, then reschedule it.

### Planning individual sessions

You are now ready to start drawing up plans for your writing slots. Think about what you want to have achieved by the end of each session. For example, you might decide to visit the library. It is not enough just to list this as one of your 'to do' activities. Write down what you want to have achieved by the end of that session. It might be to complete a database search, or to find out what books are available on a specific subject. You are almost certainly going to manage to get to the library. However, without any specific goals about what you do when you get there, you will be unable to gauge how much further on you are in your work schedule.

You may want to break tasks down into different categories. Try the following:

- planning
- writing
- research
- telephone calls
- letters
- jobs.

You may find it useful to divide your session plan into smaller squares that represent these categories.

Once you know what you want to do in the session, you can start thinking about the best order in which to do things. Arrange tasks in order of priority, starting with items that must be done in that session. If possible avoid beginning with anything that is tedious or difficult. This will only sap your energy and reduce your motivation. However, do not leave priority tasks to the end of the session, where it is likely that they might be omitted or shelved altogether. Work within your energy cycle. If you know that you tend to be sleepy after lunch, aim to carry out short tasks that are physically active, for example photocopying or filing notes. If you are brighter first thing in the morning, choose this time to do your planning and writing.

| | |
|---|---|
| Writing:<br>9.00 Draft outline for chapter four | Tel:<br>Local library re: opening times |
| 10.00 Edit typescript of chapter one | Letters:<br>Request copyright permission for diagram of lung |
| 11.00 Break | |
| Research:<br>11.20 Identify articles to follow-up at the library | |
| 12.00 Read notes from yesterday | Jobs:<br>Photocopy article on 'Respiratory Disease in Miners' at library. |
| 12.30 LUNCH | |

Figure 15.2 A daily timetable

Write out your daily goals on your timetable (see Figure 15.2). Try to achieve something every day. If you set yourself small, realistic targets it will be much more satisfying.

### Review

Monitoring of your time-management needs to be on-going and regular. This is particularly important at the beginning of a project, so you can establish a good working routine from the start. Schedule review slots for each session, day and week.

Always make a note of what you have achieved. This is an important morale booster, but will also give you some insight into what is working well for you. Think about what helped you to get a positive outcome. No distractions? Good planning? In a writing mood? Make a quick list of the factors that assisted you.

Next, look at the things that did not go to plan. Did you have uncompleted tasks? Were some items on your session plan not even attempted? Think about the factors that prevented you from achieving your goals. Did you overrun on time with some other task? Why did that happen? You may need to allow more time for some activities than you had initially anticipated. Are you using your time efficiently? Look at the section on 'Tips for Making Better Use of Your Time' below. Last, look back at the list you made on the positive factors involved with your completed goals. Use these to help in rethinking your next session.

### Tips for making better use of your time

- Be focused. Distractions and interruptions often take us away from our stated objective. Always ask yourself if what you are doing is helping you achieve your primary goals.

- Preparation and planning at the initial stages will save time later. If you lack a clear plan and structure, you are more likely to be sidetracked into irrelevant issues. Get into the habit of planning how you will use your time, and what you want to achieve within that time frame.

- Claim an area of space for yourself, and let family or flatmates know that this is your designated writing area. Always keep one surface area free of clutter. It is also useful to have storage space for your research notes, stationery and reference books like dictionaries.

○ Be organised. Make sure you have all the materials you need before you start an activity.

○ Group similar tasks together. This means you only have to find the appropriate materials or be in a certain location once, for instance planning a trip to the library so that browsing research articles can be combined with finding and returning books.

○ Give yourself 'time out' if you feel yourself getting bogged down. Alarm bells should start ringing if you find yourself rewriting a sentence dozens of times, or find it hard to assimilate information from your reading. A brisk walk or even a change in activity can bring your energy levels back up. Time away from the task is also important in promoting reflection, planning and problem-solving. Pernet (1989) describes this as an opportunity to view the situation from a 'mental helicopter'.

○ Beat procrastination:

Task seems too big – divide it into smaller subgoals, and identify the tasks required to meet these goals. It will appear, and actually be, more manageable and therefore achievable.

Task is unfamiliar – try to break the task down into smaller subgoals. You are likely to find some mini-goals that are familiar to you. Others may be achieved by adapting your knowledge and skills from other areas. For example, research skills used as a student preparing project work are easily adapted for researching material for a book. Study how others carry out activities you are unfamiliar with, or get specific help from someone who does know. For instance, librarians will offer help in carrying out database searches and libraries often run general training sessions.

Task appears daunting – use the advice for large and unfamiliar tasks. Break down into smaller steps, utilise what you know already, and plan how to find out the rest.

Task is unpleasant – what is it that makes this task unpleasant for you? Is it boring? Try spreading the task over several smaller sessions. Think about small rewards that you can give yourself when you have completed each stage.

○  Learn to say 'no'. You will always have requests, demands and pleas from others to become involved in activities that will take you away from your writing. Start thinking about time away from your writing as 'mortgaged time' (Garratt 1985). Eventually you will have to find a way of paying it back. Can you afford to do it? Set your priorities and stick by them.

○  Remember that delegation is not only for the workplace.

## Action Points

### 1. Complete an activity record

Use the activity record to record your daily activities (see Figure 15.3). Make a note of what you are doing at regular intervals. This might be as frequently as every 15 minutes or as long as an hour. Decide on the time-slots that will be of most use for you.

| **Daily Activity Record** | | |
|---|---|---|
| TIME INTERVALS | ACTIVITY | COMMENTS |
|  |  |  |
|  |  |  |
|  |  |  |
|  |  |  |
|  |  |  |
|  |  |  |
|  |  |  |
|  |  |  |
|  |  |  |
|  |  |  |
|  |  |  |
|  |  |  |
|  |  |  |
|  |  |  |

*Figure 15.3 A daily activity record*

Some activities will be lengthy and stretch over several time intervals. Others will be brief with several filling one interval. Avoid recording the minutiae of your life. Select one or two of the most important activities for recording, or alternatively use an umbrella term such as 'sorting post'.

Continue to record events on a daily basis until you have established the pattern of how you spend your time. A week is probably sufficient for most people. Remember this information is entirely for your personal use, so be honest with yourself. Write what you do, and not what you would like to do or feel you should be doing. See Figure 15.4 for an example of a completed activity record. Once this is completed, your next step is to analyse your activity records.

## Daily Activity Record

| TIME INTERVALS | ACTIVITY | COMMENTS |
|---|---|---|
| 8.30 am | Reading and sorting post | |
| 8.45 | Filing notes from yesterday's library visit | |
| 9.00 | Reading and note-taking from journal articles | |
| 9.15 | Ditto | |
| 9.30 | Ditto | |
| 9.45 | Phone calls re: car insurance | |
| 10.00 | Brainstorming outline of chapter two | |
| 10.15 | Ditto | |
| 10.30 | Went to local shops for milk | |
| | | |
| | | |
| | | |
| | | |
| | | |

*Figure 15.4 Extract from a completed daily activity record*

### 2. Making sense of the information in your activity record

Use the information in your activity record to find out what you do, when you do it and how long it takes you. This will help you see the patterns you have established in your life.

*What do I do?*

List the different activities from your record under general headings like work, home or leisure. Here are some suggestions for different categories:

- work
- social
- routine home
- personal
- hobbies/interests
- study
- writing
- family
- other obligations.

*How much time do you spend on each activity?*

Start calculating how much time is spent on each area throughout the week. If necessary you may want to further subdivide the information in each of your categories. For instance, leisure time may be divided between sports, hobbies and going to the cinema. Convert the figures to a percentage of your total available time. (This is the time between getting up in the morning and going to bed at night each day.) If you have a computer you can easily display your figures visually using graphs and pie charts. You will now have a clear idea of what you do with your time, and how much time you spend on certain activities.

*When do I do it?*

Look at the time of day that you carry out the activities. This information can be usefully displayed in the form of a Gantt chart. Place time along the horizontal axis, and activities on the vertical axis.

You might want to extend this to looking at the week as a whole. Mark the days along the horizontal axis, and the activities on the vertical axis.

Use various styles of shading to represent different activities. For instance, you can use solid shading to block out the days you are in work and cross-hatching for Saturday morning when you normally do your shopping. This type of visual display is useful for highlighting any activities that impinge on other areas. Solid shading appearing during the weekend, for example, might indicate that work-related activities were extending beyond normal contractual hours.

### Why am I doing it?

Some tasks are essential and non-negotiable. They have to be carried out. Other activities, like hobbies or seeing friends, are things that we do out of choice. How much of your time is spent on things you like to do? How much of your time is taken up with routine chores? Think about your priorities. What are the most important areas of your life? Compare this with how much time you spend on each area. Your answers may surprise you.

### 3. Find more time

Once you have completed your analysis you should have a very clear idea of how you are using your time. Are there any areas where you could be making better use of your time? You may need to do some lateral thinking. For instance, try ordering a home delivery of your groceries on the Internet. Doing a big monthly shop in this way will cut out travel and shopping time. Can you delegate any chores? You may have to enlist the help of children, partners or friends in doing some of the tasks that you would normally carry out. Is there something that you can put on hold until you have completed your project? You may have to be ruthless with yourself.

## Summary Points

○ Writing requires careful planning to ensure that you produce a quality piece of work, as well as being able to meet your deadlines.

○ Planning involves setting goals, identifying resource implications and establishing a timeframe.

○ Write down your goals for each stage of your project on a planning sheet. These will need to be further subdivided into subgoals and mini-targets.

○ Set a timeframe that accommodates your needs and allows for any other factors influencing how you manage your time.

○ Complete an activity record to find out how you are using your time at the moment. You may need to re-establish your priorities and organise your time accordingly.

○ Use your planner to draw up a timetable that includes weekly or monthly schedules covering your intended timeframe. Write out small, achievable targets for each day.

○ Monitoring of your time-management needs to be on-going and regular.

# 16

# Determining Your Style

Style is partly to do with the characteristics of the individual writer, and partly to do with the context of the written work.

Be yourself – write with your natural 'voice'. Do not try to emulate other writers or feel under pressure to create a particular style of writing.

Write for your reader – your reader's characteristics will influence your style of writing. The way in which you express yourself will alter depending on the reader's level of knowledge and experience as well as his or her attitudes and beliefs. Remember to address all your readers equally by using gender- and race-inclusive language.

Write according to your purpose – decide on your aims before you start to write. This is a key part of your planning, because without a clear purpose your writing will lack direction and structure.

Write for the situation – writing style will vary according to how and where a composition will appear. For example, a research paper requires a scientific approach whereas a magazine article might adopt a more relaxed and conversational tone.

Check your writing has an appropriate style – read your work aloud or ask a friend to review your writing and give you feedback. Thinking about the following questions will help you revise your work.

## Has it got the right tone?
### Formal versus informal
There are two main styles of writing – formal and informal. Formal writing is characterised by the use of the third person, academic terminology and objective statements. Informal writing is characterised by the use of the first person, a greater number of concrete expressions and fewer formal sentence constructions.

*Positive versus negative*

The approach to a topic might be positive or negative. The familiar saying 'Is the glass half empty or half full?' illustrates this point effectively.

*Active versus passive*

Sentences written in the active rather than the passive voice are more direct and give impact to a message. Compare 'the boy cleaned the car' (active) with 'the car was cleaned by the boy' (passive). An active sentence also gives a livelier tone to a piece of writing and tends to have fewer words. However, the use of some passive constructions is desirable to provide variety and interest for the reader.

Pitfalls:

- the use of an informal writing style in a context that requires a formal approach (and vice-versa)

- writing a piece in a tone that is inappropriate to the context (for example, most women's magazines like to take an upbeat approach to health issues)

- the use of too many passive constructions.

## Is it well structured?

Each piece of writing consists of several hierarchical layers of organisation. These range from how the overall piece is structured down to the arrangement of an individual sentence.

The whole is divided into three parts – the introduction, the middle and the end.

Groups of sentences are arranged into paragraphs. These sentences are connected by one single idea or theme, which is expanded upon throughout the paragraph.

Within each sentence, words are arranged according to their relationship to each other. For example, the verb, or doing word, is placed near to the person or thing to which it relates – so 'The dog barked.' More complex sentences are formed by a sequence of sentences known as clauses. For example, the following sentence contains two clauses: 'The dog barked but the postman was not afraid.'

Pitfalls:

- The writing lacks a clear beginning, middle or ending.

- There are too many ideas within one paragraph.

- The paragraph is overlong (usually because it contains more than one idea or theme).
- Poor sentence construction leads to ambiguity (see below).

## Does it have a logical progression?

Each paragraph within a piece will relate both to the previous paragraph and to the forthcoming one. They will all contribute to the overall theme of a composition.

Link statements help to give continuity from one paragraph to another. These sentences help explain to the reader what you are about to discuss in the new paragraph and its relationship to the previous discussion (French 1994).

The sequence in which ideas are ordered may vary. Some common ways are:

Chronological – the order follows the sequence of events as they have happened in time. (For example, a description of a client's experience of health care might be presented in a temporal sequence.)

Spatial – describes a sequence of actions. (Useful for helping the reader to visualise operations and procedures. For example, 'remove the bandage, clean the…'.)

Climactic – starts with the least important information and builds to a climax. (Useful to increase tension and anticipation.)

Defining – moves from broad concepts to specific information. (Useful for a descriptive piece.)

Analytical – looks first at the whole and then at each of the parts that make up that whole. (Useful for explanations.)

Synthesis – looks first at the small components and then combines these to form the whole. (Useful for describing solutions or problem-solving.)

Pitfalls:

- There is no connection between the ideas contained within a series of paragraphs.
- There are no link sentences to indicate a shift in topic.
- There is no logical sequence or ordering of the information.

**Is it concise?**

Make sure that your writing is succinct and to the point. Here are some tips:

- Constantly refer back to your aims whilst writing and remove any sections that are not directly relevant to your purpose.
- Use shorter words and simpler sentence structures whenever possible.
- Substitute meaningless expressions like 'now and again', 'owing to the fact that' or 'by and large' with more specific and shorter terms.
- Check for redundancies in your message, for example repetition of words that mean the same thing, as in 'erratic and irregular eating'.

**Is it interesting?**

The way that you write information can affect how interesting it is for the reader.

Try to:

- Vary the length and type of sentences.
- Vary the length of paragraphs. Lots of long paragraphs are difficult to assimilate and tiring for the reader. On the other hand, several short ones will seem repetitive and monotonous.
- Avoid repeating words, especially within the same sentence or in adjacent sentences. Use synonyms to add interest – so instead of repeatedly using personal health record, you can try 'clinical notes', 'records', 'health records' or 'notes'. (However, the use of a consistent term is recommended when writing material for clients. See Chapter 6 for more information.)
- Use action verbs. Compare the following lists:

  | complete | fill in |
  |----------|---------|
  | achieve  | do |
  | maintain | keep up |
  | compile  | put together |

○ Use words that have impact. Compare 'devastated' with 'hurt', 'sad', 'upset', 'troubled'.

## Is the meaning clear?

### *Sentence length*

Sentences that contain more than 25 words are more difficult to understand (Flesch 1964). Aim to have an average of 20 words per sentence with a maximum of three clauses.

### *Ambiguous word meanings*

There are lots of words that have more than one meaning depending on the context in which they are used. For example, the word 'sterilisation' may be a form of birth control in one situation, and a method for bacteria control in another.

Although the reader's interpretation of a word will depend on other information in the text, it is also likely to be influenced by his or her previous use of that word – so the reader may understand a word in one context but not in another. For example, 'drains' might be more familiar in relation to sewers than in relation to urinary catheters.

Select vocabulary for your reader, and use concrete terms whenever possible. These are more likely to be recognised and understood.

### *Ambiguous sentences*

Be clear when using pronouns. For example, what is the pronoun 'they' referring to in the sentence below? Is it the nurses or the clients?

> The nurses served up the patients' dinner before leaving for the staff canteen. They were very hungry.

Poor sentence construction can lead to confusions. In this example, it is unclear who has the loud voice, the doctor or the patient.

> The doctor told the patient with a loud voice about the medication.

How you use punctuation can change the meaning of a sentence entirely.

> Doctors, whose communication skills are poor, upset the clients. (This implies that all doctors have poor communication skills and upset their clients.)

Compare it with:

Doctors whose communication skills are poor upset the clients. (Only some doctors have poor communication skills, and it is these who will upset the clients.)

### Commonly confused words
Check that the words in your text are the ones you intended to use. For example:

- 'imply' (suggest) versus 'infer' (deduce)
- 'practical' (pragmatic) versus 'practicable' (feasible)
- 'less' (quantity) versus 'fewer' (number).

### The use of the apostrophe
The apostrophe (') has two functions:

1. To indicate the omission of one or more letters or numbers. For example, it's = it is and '99 = 1999.

2. To signal possession for singular and plural nouns. For example, 'the boy's bike' (singular), 'the boys' bikes' (plural). Note the apostrophe comes after the 's' in a plural noun.

Avoid common confusions that arise with the use of the apostrophe. Remember:

- 'It's' = 'it is'
  'its' = possessive, as in 'its fur'.
- Add an apostrophe and an 's' at the end of plural nouns that do not end in an 's', for example children's.

## General writing pitfalls
Here are some common pitfalls that catch most writers out at some point.

- Using clichés. These are well-known and overused words or phrases. Their use will make your writing seem hackneyed and unoriginal.
- Using inappropriate metaphors, for example, 'a growing body of evidence', 'a sea of paper' or 'a heaving sense of injustice'.
- Overstating an argument by using too many adjectives and qualifiers when describing or explaining.
- Using unnecessary jargon or reverting to colloquialisms.

## Summary Points

- Find your style by using your natural 'voice' when writing.

- Write for your reader, adjusting your style according to his or her knowledge, experience, attitudes and beliefs.

- Adapt your writing to suit different purposes and contexts.

- Style is about the structure, tone and sense of the writing.

- Simplicity and succinctness are the epitome of good style.

# 17

# Getting the Best Out of Your Personal Computer

Most writers nowadays make use of a personal computer to write and prepare their manuscript for publication. There are many advantages in terms of both cost and time. Revisions are far easier with many writing tasks automated, for example checking spelling and grammar, doing word counts. Computers with a modem also offer another mode of communication via e-mail and access to research material on the Internet.

This chapter offers an introduction to making the most of your computer as an author.

## Organising your work

### *File your work*
Create individual files for the chapters or sections of your book. Keep these in one or more folders so that you can easily locate your work. Check with your publisher's guidelines about any limits on the size of files. This is usually measured by the number of characters or words per file.

### *Database*
A database is a program that helps organise information in a similar way to a manual card index. Information such as names, addresses, dates and titles is entered onto individual records. Each of these records has a number of allotted spaces, known as fields, which contain the individual data entry. For example, one field might have the name, while another has the address. Data is easily sorted, searched and edited using the different fields. For instance, the records can be sorted to appear alphabetically, or a search carried out for all records containing the same name. A database is particularly useful for compiling bibliographies or reference lists.

## Storing your work

### Memory

Data in the form of text and graphics is stored in the memory of the computer. There are two types of memory:

- Random Access Memory (RAM) – this is the memory your computer uses to hold the text, graphics and instructions that you input as you are working on a document.

- Read Only Memory (ROM) – this is used to store information such as the programs used to run the computer.

RAM is lost when the computer is switched off. This is why you need to make sure you have saved your work, either to the hard disk (usually accessed through drive C) or onto a floppy disk (accessed through drive A).

Memory is measured in megabytes (Mb) and this is usually quoted in any specifications about a computer. It is important to check that you have sufficient memory to run the programs and store the amount of information you require. Buy the computer with the most memory you can afford.

It is a good idea to save text as you are working on a document. You need to think about how often you want to do this. For example, if you saved your work every 20 minutes, then this is the maximum amount of work you would lose if the computer crashed. Some computers have a facility where the file is automatically saved at regular time intervals. Set the time period yourself. Frequent saves mean less work will be lost if the computer suddenly crashes.

### Disks

Back up your work regularly by copying the latest version of your work onto a floppy disk. It is best to have at least two back-up disks and keep these in separate places. If one becomes lost or damaged, you then have another to replace it.

Treat your disks with respect. Find a suitable container to store them in, which will keep them free from dust and accidental damage. Avoid handling them too much.

Be methodical about how you work. Identify your current disk clearly, so that it is easily distinguishable from your back-up floppies. Label the disks using different coloured pens or labels.

Only use about three-quarters of the disk space at any one time (Dorner 1992). You will need some spare space to carry out actions like cut and paste. If the disk becomes full, the computer may be unable to complete a task and your work may be lost.

### Working with a co-author

Are you sharing a computer? If so, you need to make some decisions about how you organise your work. For instance, how will you manage joint editing? Check to see if your computer has a facility to track changes to the text. Use this to highlight edits. Alternatively, make a copy of the master document so you always have a duplicate of the original text.

Are you using different computers? The first thing to do is check whether they are compatible. If so, you can save files in ASCII (American Standard Code for Information Interchange) on a disk and share these. Make it clear which disk has the working copy (or latest agreed version) of the manuscript and which one is for back-up.

### Use your computer effectively

Use:

- Find and replace – abbreviate a lengthy name or title that you need to use frequently in your work. Use the find and replace facility to change it to the full text for your final draft.

- Spelling and grammar checker – you can install your own specialist dictionary or add to your existing one.

- Templates – set up a template for a document based on the style sheet from your publishers. For example, preset your margins and line spacing for use in new files.

- Macros – record a sequence of instructions using a single key. For instance, if you need to repeat the same piece of text or frequently format a table then use a macro. The action can be performed using one key rather than several, thus saving time.

### Be healthy

This applies to both your personal computer and yourself.

Invest in a virus checker for your computer and avoid using your disks in other machines.

Make sure that your lighting and seating is appropriate:

- Position your personal computer away from windows and direct lighting so that reflections and glare are reduced.

- ○ Have your eyesight tested regularly.
- ○ Use a proper computer chair that supports your back and encourages good posture.

Remember you will be spending many hours at your computer so being comfortable is important.

## Action Points

### *Checklist for Buying a Computer*

1. Thinking of buying a computer? Use this checklist to identify features useful for a writer.

*Writing*

- ❑ Spelling and grammar checker
- ❑ Thesaurus
- ❑ Document templates
- ❑ Macros for key words and phrases
- ❑ Alternative character sets
- ❑ Science symbols
- ❑ AutoSummarise (creates a summary)
- ❑ AutoCorrect (automatically corrects words using a preset list of errors)
- ❑ Automatic save
- ❑ Large memory.

*Editing*

- ❑ Word counts
- ❑ Find by bookmarks
- ❑ Find word and replace
- ❑ Tracking changes to text since last edit.

*Data Handling*

- ❑ Database
- ❑ Ability to convert text to ASCII.

*Printing*

- ❑ Page preview before print
- ❑ Screen shows a printed page
- ❑ Background printing
- ❑ Option on page layout.

*Hardware*

- ❑ Capacity to upgrade
- ❑ IBM compatible.

*Printer*

- ❑ Laser or bubble jet
- ❑ Fast printing speed
- ❑ Print queue capacity.

*Extras*

- ❑ CD-ROM drive
- ❑ Modem.

---

## Summary Points

- ○ Organise your work into files and folders that represent the chapters or sections of your book.
- ○ Regularly back up your work onto floppy disks.
- ○ Keep two back-up copies in case one becomes lost or damaged.
- ○ Use the computer functions to speed up your writing and editing.
- ○ Make sure you have appropriate seating and lighting when you work on your computer.

# 18

# Presenting Your Work

This chapter provides some general guidelines on the presentation and submission of written work for publication. (Completed works of this type are known as manuscripts or typescripts). Always use the following advice in conjunction with any house style rules set by your publisher.

## Paper

Use good quality A4 paper that has been designed for your particular type of printer. (Never use unbroken reels of computer paper). Type or print on one side of the paper only.

## Page layout

Allow plenty of space when you set up your margins and line spacing. The copy-editor or designer may need to use these for marking corrections or giving instructions to the typesetters.

### *Line spacing*

Lines may be single spaced, one and a half spaced or double spaced. Book manuscripts are usually double spaced. This will also apply to any text in tables, the index and captions for illustrations.

### *Margins*

Check your publisher's house style rules on the required width for margins. This will cover left, right, top and bottom margins. A standard size is usually 3 to 4 cm.

### Paragraphs

Check on indentation and line spacing for paragraphs. Requirements vary between publishers. For instance, some like to have the first line of a paragraph indented by several spaces.

### Alignment of text

Align text to the left margin. Never justify text so that spacing between words is altered to produce lines of equal length.

### Text

You must have your manuscript either typed or word-processed. Handwritten material is never acceptable.

### Font

The design of lettering will affect the readability of a manuscript. Fancy scrolls may look attractive, but make text very difficult to read. You can see the effects of different fonts in the example below:

font      **font**      font      font      fout      **font**

Choose a font with simple lettering of medium density. Remember to check that your printer is able to produce the font you are using on your computer screen. A font that appears on the screen and the printer is known as a TrueType font. Your printer manual will explain the range of fonts available to you.

### Size

The size of your lettering is also important. Choose a font size that makes the text easy to read without being overlarge. Compare the word 'font' when produced in various sizes:

Font (8)      font (10)      font (12)      font (14)

Font size 12 is easily read.

### Style

Various characteristics can be applied to lettering like italic or bold. Avoid overusing these style formats, as this can make the text confusing to read. Use any special effects judiciously and be consistent in applying them, for instance using a particular style to indicate all the main headings. Always check your publisher's house style rules, which may give specific instructions on adding style to text. Some stipulate that certain characteristics are omitted, for example using bold.

◊ Remember that your publisher will edit and prepare your work for publication. It is not your job to arrange and design the manuscript as if it were the final printed version. Your role is to prepare and present your work in a form that the editor can deal with quickly and efficiently.

## Spelling

Computers help us by providing tools that check spelling and grammar in a document. However, they are not foolproof. For example, a computer will not correct mistakes such as 'The children took their dog *fore* a walk' or 'The children took *there* dog for a walk'. Make sure you have manually checked the spelling and grammar of your final draft. This is especially important if somebody else has typed or word-processed your manuscript.

There are certain spelling conventions to which you will need to adhere. Always check your publisher's house style rules on the following:

o Variant spellings.
   Some words have alternative spellings. A common occurrence is words that can be spelt with an 's' or a 'z'. For example, the word 'specialise' can also be written as 'specialize'. Your publisher may insist on the use of one particular spelling. For instance, the use of 'z' is applicable if selling to the North American market.

o Abbreviations.
   Words are always spelt out in full, unless you want an abbreviation to appear in the final text. In that case, write out the word in full followed by the abbreviation the first time it appears in the text, for example, electronic mail (e-mail). Check whether your publisher accepts the use of common abbreviations in your manuscript, such as e.g. (for example), or requires these written in full.

o Acronyms.
   Write these out in full the first time they appear in the text, followed by the acronym in brackets. For example, urinary tract infections (UTIs).

- ○ Hyphenation.
  Be consistent about whether you hyphenate words or not.
  (Again, the publisher may stipulate that you follow one
  particular spelling rule). Do not use a hyphen to break up a
  word at the end of a line. Instead type the whole word on the
  next line down.

- ○ Proper names.
  Use a capital letter at the beginning of a proper noun (that is,
  where a name is specific to a person, place, organisation or
  object). For example, the trade name for a drug would be
  written with a capital letter, but the generic name of the same
  drug would start with a lower-case letter. (Some publications
  may insist on the use of generic names for drugs, so check
  this out.)

- ○ Names of syndromes and diseases are not usually given a
  capital letter.

- ○ Words and phrases in a foreign language.
  Check the house style rules on how to deal with accent
  marks, digraphs and Greek letters.

## Numbers

### Numerals

It is common practice to write numbers one to ten in words and those
above in figures. Alternatively you can use the rule that any number requiring more than two words should be written in figures (Winkler and
McCuen 1999).

### Percentages and amounts of money

Treat these in a similar way to numbers. The most important thing is to be
consistent in the format that you choose, and that it is acceptable to the
publisher.

### Common units of measurement

These can usually be abbreviated, for example 39°C.

### Decimal points

Place the decimal point on the line. For example, 5.0 is better than 5·0.

### Dates

A simple style is usually acceptable. For example, 26 March is better than the twenty-sixth of March or March 26th.

## Organisation

### Chapters or sections

Start each chapter of a book on a fresh sheet of paper. Titles need to match those given in your list of contents.

### Headings

Clearly indicate the difference between main headings and subheadings. Use numbers or different style characteristics to indicate the relative importance of each title. Aim for a maximum of four levels of heading.

### Lists

Indicate the relative importance of items in a list. For example, use a bold dot to represent a main point and a long dash for a minor or subpoint. Numbers and letters can also be used to list and subdivide entries.

### Page numbers

Number pages consecutively. Page numbers are usually placed in the top right-hand corner.

### Quotations

Longer quotes are usually set apart from the main text of the page, and indented from the left margin. Shorter quotations are included within the body of the text, and are enclosed by single quotation marks. (Double quotation marks are used for a quote within a quote.) Check your publisher's house style rules for specific guidance on how to present quotations.

### References

Check the style of referencing your publisher prefers, and use it consistently. Remember to make sure that any work referred to in the main text appears in your reference list. (See Chapter 12 'Dissertations' for more information on different referencing styles.)

### Cross-references

Avoid using page numbers when indicating cross-references, as these are likely to change once the manuscript is prepared for the printers. Instead refer to a particular chapter or section or use 'page 000' to indicate that a number needs to be inserted.

### *Footnotes and endnotes*

Most publishers prefer that footnotes and endnotes are kept to a minimum, so try to include as much information as possible within the main text. Type any footnotes/endnotes on separate sheets. Collate them at the end of each chapter or at the end of the manuscript. Remember to indicate their intended position in the text by using an appropriate symbol like an asterisk, number or letter.

## Tables, figures and illustrations

You may want to use some form of visual material to support your text, for example graphs, figures, drawings and photographs.

Always discuss the use of illustrations with your publisher before you spend time and money on producing items. Certain forms of illustration are very costly for the printers to reproduce, and may either be rejected or the expense passed on to you as the author. Some publishers also prefer to use an in-house illustrator, or are able to buy in suitable material that has been professionally produced.

Use the following guidelines in conjunction with advice from your publisher on how to prepare and submit visual material.

- Make sure your illustrations are clear and accurate.

- Avoid using illustrations as decoration. Only use visual material that is essential for explaining and supporting the information in your text.

- Aim to prepare material to a professional standard.

- Keep illustrations as simple as possible. Any graphics you submit must be in a form that can be easily reproduced by the printers of the book or journal.

- Check the size of the original material with the size of the printed page. Remember that once your illustration has been reduced to fit the size of the book or journal page much of the detail may be lost.

- Present each illustration on a separate page.

- Remember to include any captions, titles and references to or acknowledgements of permission to quote material. Captions should include any references to parts of the illustration, for example, A – outer ear, B – middle ear, and C – inner ear.

○ Provide an explanation of any symbols.

○ Check that all spellings and abbreviations are consistent with those in the main text.

○ Collate your illustrations either at the end of a chapter or at the end of your manuscript.

○ Make sure you have put some identification information on the back of any illustrations, for example your name (and any co-author's name), the title of the manuscript, any captions, and a number (see below) that indicates the order in which they appear in the text. It is often better to do this in pencil so marks will not show through onto the drawing or artwork. An alternative is to photocopy material and mark it with the appropriate information.

○ Remember to mark which side is the 'top' of the illustration as this will not always be clear to a non-health professional.

○ Number your illustrations so that the publisher is able to identify where and in what order items will appear in the text. For example, the first table in Chapter 2 would be numbered 2.1, the next 2.2 and so on. Mark the position in the main body of the text by typing 'insert Table 2.1 here'. Use these numbers when making references to these items in the main text, for example, 'see Table 2.1' or 'see Figure 5.2' (Do not include page numbers as these will change once the manuscript has been typeset.)

## Submitting your work
### Hard copy
This term refers to a printed or typed manuscript. Publishers usually require two copies if no electronic copy is supplied. Always retain a third copy for yourself.

Arrange the order of your manuscript according to your publisher's guidelines with the pages loose. Do not use paper clips or treasury tags to fasten them together. Insert a cover sheet with your name, contact details and the title of your manuscript.

### *Electronic copy*

It is common practice for publishers to request an electronic copy of a manuscript in the form of text stored on disk. One printed or typed version of the manuscript is usually submitted with an electronic copy. The information on your disk must be identical to this hard copy.

Check your publisher's guidelines on how to submit electronic versions of your manuscript. The most important point to consider is whether the publisher's computer will be able to read your disk. Find out the specifications on:

- the type of hardware
- the type of word-processing package(s)
- the type, size and density of disk.

(It may be worth submitting a trial disk at the beginning of your project.)

You will almost certainly be asked to convert your documents to plain text or ASCII. Use one file per chapter, and make a separate file for graphics. Some computer commands are difficult to translate and you may be given specific instructions about the preparation of your files.

Label each disk clearly with your name and the title of the manuscript, and include a list of the files. Mark the type and density of the disk if not already apparent. Some publishers also like to have the details of the name of your computer and the word-processing package you have used to prepare the disk. Remember to keep a copy on disk for yourself.

### Packaging

Package your printed manuscript and disks with care. Just think of the effort and the cost involved in replacing them if they get lost or damaged in the post. The postal system can be a rough-and-tumble experience for packages. An ordinary envelope containing a heavy item like a manuscript is more at risk of ripping and spilling out its contents. Use reinforced envelopes like padded bags or place the manuscript in a cardboard box and send it as a parcel. Include a cover sheet with your name and contact details in case there is any mishap in the post.

## Action Points
### *Checklist for presenting your manuscript*

*Paper*

- ❑ A4 paper
- ❑ Printed one side only.

*Page layout*

- ❑ Margins set at...
- ❑ All lines are.........spaced
- ❑ Text is aligned with the left-hand margin.

*Text*

- ❑ Font...
- ❑ Font size...
- ❑ Style effects have been kept to a minimum and used consistently.

*Spelling*

- ❑ Spelling and grammar check is completed
- ❑ Spelling conventions comply with the house style of the publisher
- ❑ Choice of variant spellings is consistent.

*Quotations*

- ❑ Copyright permission is enclosed for lengthy quotations
- ❑ Lengthy quotes are set apart from the main text of the page, and indented from the left margin
- ❑ Shorter quotations have been included within the body of the text, and are enclosed by quotation marks.

*References*

- ❑ References cited in the text agree with those listed in your reference list

❑ Reference list is presented in a format acceptable to the publisher.

*Illustrations*

❑ All tables, figures and artwork have been submitted in the agreed format

❑ Each one has been numbered and labelled

❑ Position has been indicated in the body of the main text

❑ Written permission on copyright material is enclosed where necessary.

*Organisation*

❑ Each chapter starts on a new page

❑ Pages are numbered consecutively in the top right-hand corner

❑ The manuscript is arranged in the order requested by the publisher.

*Submission*

❑ One or two printed copies for publisher

❑ One copy in plain text or ASCII on disk for publisher

❑ Each disk has been labelled with your name and the title of the manuscript

❑ One copy on disk for yourself

❑ One printed version for yourself.

## Summary Points

○ Manuscripts must be typed or printed on one side of A4 paper.

○ Text needs to be well spaced with clear and simple lettering. Keep style effects to a minimum, and be consistent in how you use them.

○ Check spelling and grammar. Make sure you comply with the house style rules of the publisher.

○ Always discuss the use of illustrations with the publisher before you spend any time or money on producing materials.

○ Copies submitted on disk must be saved in plain text or ASCII. Keep chapters and graphics in separate files.

○ Carefully package manuscripts for posting in a protective envelope or cardboard box.

○ Always retain at least one copy on disk and one printed version for yourself.

# 19

# Protecting Your Rights

This chapter looks at the two main ways of protecting the author's rights – the law on copyright and the publishing contract. It is not meant to be a definitive account, and the reader is advised to refer to the relevant legislation. Always seek legal advice if you are in any doubt about copyright or contractual matters.

◊ What is the law on copyright?

The Copyright, Designs and Patents Act of 1988 provides, amongst other things, protection for original literary works and the typographical arrangements of published editions.

It is useful for authors to note that copyright applies to the form in which ideas are expressed, and not to the ideas themselves. Copyright does not subsist in the literary work until it is recorded in writing or other similar means. However, it is not necessary for the work to be published.

◊ Who owns the copyright?

In general this is usually the author. However, if the author has completed the work as part of his or her duties as an employee, then the employer has ownership. The author may also assign copyright to the publisher, a common practice when work is published in journals. In these cases authors who try to resell an article, without the permission of the journal's publisher, will infringe copyright law.

◊ What is the term of copyright ownership?

In the United Kingdom, copyright is usually the life of the author plus 70 years. Copyright for the typographical arrangement of a published edition expires at the end of 25 years. However, there are variations in copyright, especially between countries, so never assume that copyright has expired. Always check first.

◊ When do I need to get permission?

You need to get permission to reproduce original or adapted versions of the following:

1. Illustrations such as photographs, figures, drawings, graphs and tables.

2. Single quotations of more than 300 words or several quotations from the same source that are equivalent to more than 300 words (Churchill Livingstone 1996).

However, it should be noted that the Act states that 'substantial parts of the work' are measured in terms of *quality* and not *quantity*, so use the above word limit with caution. Seek the advice of your publisher or contact the copyright owner if you are unsure.

You will need to acknowledge the original source of any copyrighted material you use in your own work. Indicate the granting of permission within the text of your work, for example, 'Reproduced with the kind permission of...'.

◊ How do I get permission?

Write to the copyright holder to obtain written permission for using material. Give precise details of what you want to copy, for example the title of the work and the page and line numbers. Explain why you want to use the work and give assurance that the author or copyright owner will be acknowledged. You may be charged a fee. Send a copy or copies of this written permission to the publisher with your completed manuscript.

◊ How does the copyright law affect photocopying?

There are restrictions on the photocopying of copyright material. You may legitimately make a single copy of written material for private study or research. However, this must be no more than 5 per cent of the whole work, for example a single chapter. If you are copying an article from a journal you may only copy one item from that issue. There are some exceptions to these rules; for instance, an educational institution may be licensed by the Copyright Licensing Agency to make multiple copies if these are for use in class.

## Contracts

Contracts between an author and publisher are usually known as a 'publishing agreement' or 'memorandum of agreement'.

### *Journal articles*

An author will be asked to sign an agreement when his or her manuscript has been accepted for publication. It will contain information on:

- the content of the article
- the word length
- the date for delivery of the manuscript
- presentation of the manuscript
- methods and amount of payment.

### *Books*

An author will be asked to sign an agreement once his or her proposal has been accepted. It is not necessary to have completed the whole manuscript. In fact it is probably unwise to continue with a writing project without such an agreement.

Contracts will usually contain information on the following items:

- rights granted to the publisher (the right to publish the work and the territories)
- subsidiary rights (for example, translation and electronic rights)
- author's warranty (for example, work is original, copyright permission obtained where necessary)
- presentation of the manuscript (for instance, use of disks, number of hard copies)
- date of delivery of manuscript (your deadline)
- date of publication (usually 12 to 18 months after the date of delivery)
- method and amount of payment (including accountancy dates)
- proofs and author's liability for corrections

- copyright (confirmation that the author's name will appear with due prominence along with the copyright notice)
- index (relates to payment for professional indexer if required)
- illustrations (again relates to conditions when payment might be necessary)
- author's liability to revise
- author's copies (authors are usually allowed between 4 to 6 free copies)
- termination (circumstances under which the contract might be terminated).

## Payment

There are two main forms of payment – 1. a single lump sum payment and 2. royalties.

1. A one-off payment is usually made for journal articles, although it is also a perfectly feasible method of payment for a book. The amount is set by the publisher and agreed with the author via a publishing agreement. The payment is usually received a few months after publication and is not affected by the amount of subsequent sales.

2. Royalties are paid as a percentage of the net sales receipts received by the publisher from the sale of the book. An average figure for a single author book is 10 per cent, but authors will find that royalties may be lower or higher than this figure. This will depend on the publisher, the type of book and the author. For instance, a well-known and popular author will be able to command a higher royalty percentage. Most publishers will have a six-month accounting period with payments made twice a year (three months after the end of each accounting period).

The above payments should be distinguished from payments known as advances. These sums are usually paid in advance of publication against future royalty payments – so if you receive an advance of £500, it will be deducted from your first royalty payment.

Always check the contract carefully and seek legal advice if in doubt about any part of the agreement.

## Summary Points

° The Copyright, Designs and Patents Act of 1988 provides, amongst other things, protection for original literary works and the typographical arrangements of published editions.

° Copyright applies to the form in which ideas are expressed, and not to the ideas themselves.

° The author usually has ownership of copyright. In some circumstances, ownership may belong to an employer or be assigned to the publisher.

° Contracts between an author and publisher are usually known as a 'publishing agreement' or 'memorandum of agreement'.

° There are two main forms of payment. A single lump sum payment is usually made for articles. Royalties, a percentage of the net sales, are the more common method of payment for books.

# 20

# Publication Skills in Context
## Journal Articles

Health journals are one of the main forms of communication both within and between the health disciplines. They provide a forum for disseminating information, sharing ideas and initiating debate. Most journals are published monthly or quarterly, and offer readers a relatively up-to-date source of information.

Journals vary in the type of articles they publish. Some only accept research papers, while others are looking for more general features on clinical and professional issues. Topics range from clinical practice, medical education and health management to more general professional concerns.

### Why write a journal article?

There are many professional and personal reasons that prompt clinicians to write articles. You will find the many benefits include the following.

- Personal development through:
  - furthering your understanding of your chosen topic
  - developing your writing skills
  - receiving validation of your work through peer review.
- Improving client care by:
  - sharing your knowledge and expertise
  - passing on best practice
  - highlighting new developments
  - increasing awareness of innovations.
- Supporting the process of continuing education by:
  - helping clinicians apply theory to practice

- sharing skills and expertise
- highlighting issues for debate
- providing an update on clinical practice.
- Contributing to the evidence base for clinical practice by:
  - disseminating your research findings
  - reporting on the application of theory to practice
  - challenging existing beliefs.
- Enhancing your career by:
  - gaining kudos from having your work published
  - increasing your academic or professional credibility.

**What do you write?**

Journals offer clinicians an opportunity to write using a range of styles and approaches. Types of articles regularly seen in journals include:

- research papers
- literature reviews
- case studies
- debates and discussions
- opinion pieces (clinical, professional, managerial or topical)
- features on special projects
- examples of best practice (clinical, managerial or organisational)
- clinical education (for example, new methods of assessing students)
- professional issues (for example, giving presentations)
- innovations or new initiatives
- clinical updates.

**Finding the right journal**

You are more likely to be successful if you write your article with a particular journal in mind. Your choice of publication will be based on a number of factors.

### 1. Your reading habits

Most clinicians choose to submit their articles to a journal which they regularly subscribe to or read (White 1987). However, you may find it worth your while to consider a range of journals, both those that are read by your discipline and those of other health professionals.

What journals do you regularly read? Are they the most suitable ones for your type and style of article? What other journals might be suitable?

### 2. Your reason for writing an article

You may be influenced in your choice of a journal by your reasons for writing your article. For example, academics working in a higher education institution are expected to publish research. Their first choice for publishing a research paper would be a peer-reviewed journal. Alternatively, a clinician who wants to share an example of best practice with other professionals might submit it to a journal with a multidisciplinary readership.

Why are you writing your article? How might your reasons influence your choice of journals?

### 3. Your target audience

Be specific about your intended readers. Identify the discipline or disciplines who would be interested in reading your article.

Which journal or journals do they usually read?

### 4. Your choice of topic

Journals usually have a clear idea about the type of subject matter that they are seeking from contributors. Some are interested in articles dealing with a particular clinical speciality; others are looking for material that would be of interest to a specific discipline. There are also journals that focus on more general areas such as management, clinical education or certain types of intervention.

Is your topic suitable for your target journal? Find out by reading several back issues and studying the guidelines for contributors.

### 5. Your style and approach

It is important to match the journal's usual style, approach and word limit when writing your article.

Will your article conform to the journal's format?

Research your target journal thoroughly. It will help if you know:

- ○ the journal's target readership
- ○ how often it is published
- ○ the ethos of the journal
- ○ the type of articles
- ○ the general approach of the journal
- ○ the style of presentation
- ○ the journal's usual contributors (there may be restrictions).

Once you have identified a suitable journal, you can start to develop your ideas about your article. See below on 'Writing your journal article' for more information.

### Approaching a journal

You may want to consider discussing your idea with the editor before you write your article. Using a query letter is one way of doing this. See Chapter 22 'Articles for the Media' for more information. Whether you are writing a letter or sending the whole manuscript, only approach one journal at a time. If the editor knows that you have contacted other journals, he or she is almost certain to reject your article.

Many journals have specially appointed experts who assess submissions. This is usually a 'double-blind' review, so that the reviewer and author are not told each other's names. These reviewers where necessary will make suggestions about revisions, to either the content or the format of articles.

You may be lucky and have your article accepted without the need for changes. However, it is not uncommon for revisions to be requested before an article is accepted, so do not be alarmed if your work is returned with a request for a rewrite. You will need to resubmit your article once you have made the revisions. Discuss any queries about this with the editor.

Unfortunately you may receive a firm 'no, thank you'. Most journals will try to give some feedback on why your article has been rejected. However, some decline to do this, and all will refuse to engage in any on-going debates. Depending on the feedback, you may want to submit your article to another journal.

### Writing your journal article

Your choice of topic will be affected by your interests and expertise. It is easier to write on a subject about which you are very knowledgeable and that arouses your keen interest. You may also want to take the advice of the editor who may have a particular theme in mind for future editions.

### Planning your article

#### Consider your aims

The first step in planning your article is to decide on your overall aim. What do you want to achieve with your article?

| **Aim**: | **Outcome**: |
|---|---|
| To *teach* a skill | Reader *learns* a skill |

How will your article help your reader learn a skill? You might want to give a sequence of instructions, explanations and practical examples. Do you need illustrations?

| | |
|---|---|
| To *share* innovative or best practice | Reader *is able to apply principles or model to own practice* |

Check that your approach is innovative by researching information about current practices. Have you proof that your model benefits your clients, service or organisation?

| | |
|---|---|
| To explain or *provide an update* on theory | Reader *increases knowledge* and *understanding* |

Engage your reader with the material by suggesting ways of following up theory through independent study, real life experiences and by providing self-assessment exercises. Most journals will prefer that the theoretical aspects of your article are related to clinical practice.

| | |
|---|---|
| To *challenge* or *stimulate* debate | Reader *thinks, reflects* or *challenges back*! |

Choose a controversial issue, challenge a traditional belief or take an unusual perspective on a topic. However, remember to support your arguments with facts, figures and examples.

| | |
|---|---|
| To *disseminate* research | Reader *increases knowledge of evidence base* and *applies findings to practice* |

Journals will be particularly interested in the results of your research and their implications for clinical practice.

To *identify issues* of importance             Reader has greater *awareness*

These articles highlight issues that the reader has not yet had time to consider or may have limited knowledge about. For example, you might want to write about the implications of a new piece of legislation for clinical practice.

To *entertain*                          Reader *enjoys*

Some journals accept items that are purely for the entertainment of the reader rather than for any academic or professional reason. A humorous piece, a collection of anecdotes or a historical piece, are just some examples. These types of articles are often written in the first person.

Be clear about the basic theme of your article. Once you are sure of this yourself it will be much easier to communicate it to your reader. Write out the purpose of your article in one sentence. Redraft it until you think you have a clear and succinct statement, for example, 'to explain the signs and symptoms of depression, its causes, traditional classifications and management options'.

*Consider your target readership*

- ○ What do they know already? – think about the reader's existing knowledge and experience of your topic area.
- ○ What do they need to know? – think about your aims and what you would like your article to achieve.
- ○ How will they use your information? – think about practical applications.

Answering these questions is particularly important if you are writing an article for members of another discipline. For example, an occupational therapist writing an article on poor hand–eye co-ordination for teachers will need to think carefully about the knowledge base of his or her readers.

Add your target audience to your statement of purpose, for example, 'explain to district nurses the signs and symptoms of depression, its causes, traditional classifications and management options'.

*Decide on the content*

Your statement of purpose or your objective forms the starting point for drafting the content of your article. Brainstorming using the keywords from your objective is a useful way of developing ideas. It may help this process if you set yourself a series of questions. In the above example, you might want to ask some of the following questions. What is depression? Why do people become depressed? What are the physical symptoms? What are the affective symptoms? How is depression treated? How do we distinguish between the different types of depression?

The key areas or concepts identified through this process will form your section headings. Even if these are not used as titles in the final article, they can act as markers for how you will organise your material.

### Creating a structure

Forming a structure early on in your planning will help in refining your search for information. Here are some examples of different formats for presenting material in articles.

#### Research papers

Research articles or research papers are always written using the traditional scientific approach discussed in Chapter 13 'Research Projects'. An example of a quantitative research paper is the abstract. An abstract consists of a short paragraph that summarises the research paper for the reader. It is placed at the beginning of an article. Most are 200 to 250 words in length, although some journals may accept longer ones.

A reader can use the abstract to quickly make a decision about whether the research findings are of relevance to him or her and therefore worth reading. On a database, an abstract may be the only information available to the searcher on the contents of a paper.

Abstracts contain:

- a statement about the purpose of your research
- your hypothesis or your research question
- a description of your research design
- your rationale for choosing that design
- a statement about your methods and procedures that includes details of any special equipment and the selection and number of subjects
- a description of your data analysis
- your major findings
- your conclusions

> ○ implications for further research or applications to practice.

The organisation of the abstract very much reflects the structure of the research paper, the standard format being:

> ○ Introduction (this contains information about relevant literature, the purpose and rationale for your research and your hypothesis)
>
> ○ Methods
>
> ○ Results
>
> ○ Discussion of results
>
> ○ Conclusion.

### Other formats

Example of a literature review:

> ○ Introduction (reason for or objectives in conducting the review)
>
> ○ Rationale for literature selection
>
> ○ Critical analysis of the literature
>
> ○ Results of your review
>
> ○ Conclusions
>
> ○ Implications for further research
>
> ○ Applications to clinical practice.

Example of a clinical update on skin diseases:

> ○ Incidence of skin diseases
>
> ○ Description of skin
>
> ○ Effect on client (psychological aspects, physical factors, quality of life)
>
> ○ Assessment (including a description of different skin diseases)
>
> ○ Treatment
>
> ○ Summary (a position statement).

Example of a debate on clinical supervision:

> ○ Introduction (definition of clinical supervision, statement on the purpose and terms of reference of the article)

- Overview of the models of supervision
- Comparison of models of delivery
- Discussion of the benefits of supervision (supported by references to research).

Example of a continuing professional development article on 'depression':

- Statement about the aims and intended learning outcomes for the reader, for example:
  - describe the signs and symptoms of depression
  - list common causes of depression
  - differentiate between the four classifications of depression
  - describe four treatments for depression
- Introduction
- Definition of depression
- Common causes
- Signs and symptoms
- Classification of depression
- Treatments
- Conclusion (applications to practice).

A teaching article of this sort might suggest other complementary forms of study. In the above example, the reader might be asked to reflect on his or her own experience of depression, complete a self-assessment questionnaire on the basic facts, and make a list of symptoms noted in a client diagnosed with depression.

A well-structured article will be organised and logical, and will only include information that is necessary to meet your aims.

### Researching your article
Your next step is to carry out a thorough literature review of your intended subject area. This will help you in gauging the current level of knowledge. See Chapter 7 'Writing As an Aid to Learning' for information on searches.

### Writing your draft
Your approach and style will very much depend on your readership. When you are writing an article for colleagues within your own discipline you

will be able to assume a certain knowledge base. It will be appropriate to use well-known terminology without the need for extensive explanations. However, other groups of readers, despite being a professional audience, will not always have a specialist knowledge of your subject area. You will need to take this into account when introducing information and in your use of terminology.

Be careful not to make your subject area too wide, as you must comply with the word limit set by the journal. Set yourself limits so that you are able to deal effectively with the information within the constraints of a short article. Constantly refer back to your objective to keep you on track with your task.

### *Editing your draft*
Careful editing of your article is essential. Double-check the accuracy of facts and figures, particular the dosage for drugs. Continually monitor events so that your information remains as up-to-date as possible.

## References
Some journals place a limit on the number of references per article and this is often an indication of the academic level they are seeking. There are two commonly used styles of referencing – the Harvard and the Vancouver. Always check the journal's guidelines for contributors on exactly how to present your references. See Chapter 12 'Dissertations' for more information.

## Formalities
Follow your organisation's protocol on publication and seek permission for an article that relates in any way to your employment, for example if you have developed a procedure through work or your organisation is identified in the article.

Remember to protect the confidentiality of clients. For example, names and details can be changed in case studies.

## Presentation and submission of your journal article
Journals usually require articles to be submitted on disk with one or two printed copies. Send these to the appropriate editor with a covering letter that includes your name and contact details. Never e-mail or fax your article.

It is important that you conform to the journal's guidelines for contributors. These will give you information about page layout, style and format. Journals usually require graphics to be presented on a separate disk and may limit the type and number of illustrations. (See Chapter 18 'Presenting Your Work' for more general advice on presentation of manuscripts.)

You may or may not be sent proofs for checking. These are print-outs that show how the article will actually look on the journal page. This is not the time to rewrite your article; only amend technical or copyright errors. You may have to pay for any other changes. Return the proofs by the agreed deadline, otherwise you may find the article goes to print containing the unamended errors.

**Action Points**

***Checklist for reviewing your article***

1. Setting up a peer review group is a useful way for potential authors to offer a critique on each other's work. Use this checklist to help provide feedback to each other.

*General*

- ❑ Is it current?
- ❑ Is it interesting? Why?
- ❑ Is it original?
- ❑ Has it got relevance or importance for clinical practice?

*Style*

- ❑ Is it at an appropriate level for the reader?
- ❑ Has unnecessary jargon been avoided?
- ❑ Is terminology explained?

*Topic*

- ❑ Is it relevant to the intended reader?
- ❑ Is it appropriate for the target journal?
- ❑ Does the article provide comprehensive coverage of the topic or are there gaps?
- ❑ Has it got practical applications?

*Efficacy*

- ❑ Is there evidence to support the author's claims or statements?
- ❑ Is reference made to other work?
- ❑ Does the data or technical information quoted in the article support or contradict the author's conclusions?

*Writing style*

- ❑ Does the content relate to the title?
- ❑ Does the content relate to the stated aims of the article?
- ❑ Are arguments developed in a logical way?
- ❑ Does the text flow or does it seem disjointed?
- ❑ Is it clear? If not, why?

*Format*

- ❑ Does the length conform to the journal's specifications?
- ❑ Is the length appropriate to meet the aims of the article?
- ❑ Is the technical information accurate?
- ❑ Are diagrams and tables complete?
- ❑ Does it conform to the target journal's guidelines for submission?

*References*

- ❑ Are they relevant?
- ❑ Are they accurate?
- ❑ Do references in the text agree with those in the reference list?
- ❑ Do they conform to the journal's guidelines?
- ❑ Do they reflect current research and opinion?

## Summary Points

- Health journals offer a forum for disseminating information, sharing ideas and initiating debate.

- You are more likely to be successful if you write your article with a particular journal in mind.

- The first step in planning your article is to decide on your overall aim. Write a clear and succinct statement about the purpose of your article.

- Creating a structure for your article early on in your planning will help in refining your search and planning your writing.

- Many journals have specially appointed experts who assess submissions. It is not uncommon for revisions to be requested before an article is accepted.

- Remember to seek permission for an article that relates in any way to your employment.

- Always protect the confidentiality of clients.

# 21

# Books

Writing a book is a great personal and professional achievement. It also provides the opportunity:

- to complete a large scale piece of writing
- to write about your subject at length and in detail
- to reach a wider audience than that offered through other writing forums
- to satisfy a creative urge.

**Developing an idea**

Before approaching a publisher you will need to have formulated some preliminary ideas about:

- the topic or specific subject area
- the aims of your book
- the scope of your book
- the intended readership
- your style or approach (is it an academic text, practical guide, directory, handbook or one that combines text with a CD-ROM?).

Chapter 14 'Developing an Idea' offers more suggestions about how to develop an idea for writing.

## Single author or collaborative writing?

At this stage you may also want to think about whether you want to write the book yourself or share the task with one or more other authors. There are advantages and disadvantages to both these methods of working.

As a single author you:

o  receive sole credit

o  have control over the decision making

o  are able to work at your own pace

o  need to make fewer compromises.

The downside is:

o  it is more work

o  you have sole responsibility

o  you miss out on the enthusiasm and support you gain from having a writing partner(s).

In collaborative writing you are able:

o  to generate new ideas between you

o  to share the workload

o  to give and receive support and encouragement

o  to benefit from different perspectives.

The downside is you will need:

o  to negotiate with your partner(s), which may mean having to make compromises

o  to combine different writing styles and ways of working

o  to make time for meetings and joint planning

o  to organise the sharing of a working manuscript.

If you do choose to work with someone else you will need to make a decision about who will be the lead author. This is necessary, as the publisher will prefer to deal with one person who is able to represent everyone's views.

**Is there a market?**

You need to think very carefully about whether there is a market for your idea. Your topic may be your lifetime passion, but is it of interest to other people? It must have sufficient readership to make it worth publishing.

Discussions with colleagues, particularly those involved in education, will help to highlight the current trends in reading material. Find out about the latest books on the market. You can do a literature search or ask advice from a librarian who is a specialist in your area. Most publishers also provide information on books that they are planning to publish in the coming year.

Study complementary or competitive texts to check that your idea is new or different in some way from other publications. Think about how your book will differ from these texts:

- Do you have a new or different concept, for example an innovative clinical approach?

- Are you thinking of a new or different format, for example, combining the traditional text of a book with a CD-ROM?

- Have you got a new or different perspective on a topic, for example a critique of written client information using feedback and comments from clients themselves?

- Is your book a response to current changes in legislation or health care provision?

**Approaching a publisher**

Unless you have been lucky enough to have been asked to write something by a commissioning editor, you will have to make the first approach. Once you have a firm idea about the book you would like to write, start looking for a suitable publisher. You need one that deals with your subject area and has access to the appropriate markets for your book.

Find out the names of publishers and the types of books they publish by checking what is currently on the market. You can access this information through a variety of sources including:

- libraries

- bookshops

- catalogues

- ○ journals
- ○ book exhibitions at various conferences
- ○ World Wide Web.

Information about publishers can also be found in the following guides:

- ○ *The Writer's Handbook*
- ○ *Willings Press Guide*
- ○ *Writers' & Artists' Yearbook.*

Some publishers have pre-prepared sheets offering advice and information to prospective writers. An alternative to this official statement is the views of friends or colleagues who have been published by them. These will give you invaluable insight into your likely experiences with them as an author. Librarians are another excellent source of information.

Remember to consider the design of the books as well as their content. Does the publisher mainly produce academic texts? Or does it concentrate on practical resources like handbooks and self-help guides? The format of books is especially important if you have a specific style in mind, for instance if you want to provide a practical guide for parents using sheets that can be photocopied.

Make a list of suitable publishers but only approach one at a time. Your initial contact is probably best made through a query letter giving brief information about yourself that includes your qualifications and any writing experience. Do not be concerned if this is your first book, as previous publications are not an essential requirement. However, it may be useful to highlight any substantial writing projects that you have completed. For example, writing a dissertation for a higher degree or preparing a service development plan will show your commitment and ability to deliver a substantial piece of work.

Your letter should be accompanied by a synopsis of your book that outlines its aims, approach and content. Include details on the type of reader you expect to buy your book. The letter needs to be sent to the commissioning editor, who will take it to an editorial meeting for discussion.

### Writing a proposal

At some stage the publisher is likely to ask for a full proposal in writing, so it is worth putting together information as soon as possible.

A proposal will usually contain the following:

1.  A description of the book with an outline of the contents

2.  A statement about your reasons for writing the book

3.  The target market or readership

4.  A review of competing or complementary texts

5.  The estimated timeframe

6.  Places to market.

### 1. A description of the book (see 'Writing your book' below)

Start with a statement that describes the aims, scope, style and approach of the book. For example: 'This is a handbook for student physiotherapists on how to write a research paper. It aims to provide a review of the current approaches to writing both quantitative and qualitative research papers. It provides self-learning exercises, examples and explanatory notes.' Here the aim of the book is matched by its style (a practical study text) – an approach designed to attract the interest of its intended audience.

Give an outline of the contents. List the chapters or sections with a brief description of the content. You may be able to change this later, but this must be before the publisher starts preparing any advertising material for catalogues or fliers – so try to be clear about what you want to include in the book and in what order you want to arrange it.

Indicate the length of your book. This is traditionally measured by the number of words rather than the number of pages or chapters. Although this is an estimation, it is important to be as accurate as possible. Aim for your final manuscript to be at least within 5000 words of your agreed limit.

### 2. A statement about your reasons for writing the book

A few lines about your personal reasons for writing the book will add interest to your proposal. This section is not just about your personal motivation. It is also an opportunity to sell both yourself and your ideas. For instance, you may have a desire to share your many years of experience with students just starting out in your profession. This is a good reason for writing a book, but it also highlights your expertise. You are somebody with something to offer. Alternatively, there may be specific events that have prompted you to consider writing a book, for example changes in legislation or new developments in clinical practice. Outline these and indicate how they relate to your book.

### 3. The target market or readership

The publisher will find it helpful to know exactly who you think will read your book. Consider the different markets available to you:

◊ The primary market
The primary market consists of those readers who will form the majority of your intended audience. Be specific about exactly who your book is aimed at.

◊ Secondary markets
Are there any other groups of readers who may be interested in your book? These readers will form your secondary markets. For example, a book aimed at district nurses might also be useful for other types of community nurses.

◊ International markets
Do you think your book will be read in other countries? This will very much depend on the content and whether it is transferable between different cultures and languages.

◊ Further and higher education
Is your book likely to be a useful text for a training course? If so, state the name of the course and an estimate of the likely number of students.

### 4. A review of competing or complementary texts

You will need to do some research in order to offer a critique of other books that are similar to your own in content, style or approach. Check the competition to see whether they are:

   ○ out of date

   ○ directed at a different market, for example postgraduates rather than undergraduates

   ○ written in a different style, for example academic versus practical

   ○ set at a different level, for example introductory versus advanced

- ○ different in the range and depth of their contents, for example a general text on obstetric procedures compared with a comprehensive and in-depth study of episiotomy

- ○ relevant only to a specific health care system or country, for example a book for nurse practitioners working in the UK.

Select a few key texts that might rival your own and write a brief review. Point out the reasons why your book will offer something different and thus address a gap in the market.

### 5. The estimated timeframe

You will need to agree a date with the publisher for submission of your completed manuscript. Before you start any negotiations, be clear about exactly how much time you require to write your book. This will depend on a number of factors:

- ○ how fast or slow you are at the actual writing process

- ○ the specific demands of the task (Do you need to do a lot of research? Are you collecting together resource ideas?)

- ○ the length and complexity of the contents

- ○ the style of the book (extra time may be required at the design stage for illustrations or unusual page layouts).

Plan time for preparing the manuscript for the publishers as this can be more time-consuming than you think. Remember you will also have some work to do after submission, for example responding to queries from the editor and checking the manuscript once it is typeset. The publisher will also have an on-going schedule and will need to arrange a slot for preparing your manuscript for the printers. This will often be at least 18 months or more from the acceptance of your original proposal.

If your book is linked to current events you may need to identify a publisher who can give you a swift turnaround time – therefore it is a good idea to establish with the publisher whether the timeframe is feasible before you enter any agreements.

### 6. Places to market

Make a list of journals, conferences and so on where the publisher will be able to advertise your book.

**Submitting your proposal**

Remember to take care when presenting your proposal. You are selling yourself as well as your book. Make sure that it is accurate and professionally presented. Check that you have included enough detail to convince the publishers to commit time and effort to your idea.

It is hoped that you will be in the happy position of having your proposal accepted and you can agree terms. See Chapter 19 on 'Protecting Your Rights' for information on contracts.

Be prepared for a rejection of your idea. If this does happen, make sure that you get some feedback from the commissioning editor. They may already have a similar book scheduled or feel the topic is unsuitable for their market. Frank discussion may generate some ideas about how to modify your proposal or provide names of other publishers who may be more interested in your book. Most editors are usually very helpful when dealing with submissions.

**Writing your book**

There is nothing mystical about writing a book. It follows the same steps as any other piece of writing:

- planning
- research
- writing
- editing
- preparation of the final draft.

The main feature that distinguishes writing a book from any other type of composition is the sheer amount of work involved. Books usually require more in-depth research, as you are unlikely to be able to write one solely from experience or your current knowledge. For instance, academic texts require detailed references to current research and theories. Be prepared to deal with a large quantity of information that may be complex in nature. There is a surprising amount of work even in non-academic texts. These are all things you need to consider carefully before committing yourself to the task.

You will have made a plan as part of preparing your proposal. This will have helped you in identifying the:

- ○ What? – your topic and its scope
- ○ Who? – your target readers
- ○ Why? – your purpose or what you intend to achieve with the book
- ○ How? – your approach will depend on the answers to the above questions.

Traditional brainstorming techniques work well when you are trying to establish the contents for a book. Identifying key points in this way often helps to formulate chapter or section headings. Once you have these you are more able to think about the most appropriate sequence for the contents.

Study how different authors have organised the contents of their books. You will find that some subjects have a natural sequence. For example, a midwifery book might start at conception, move through pregnancy and finish with birth. Other subject matter may need to be approached in a different way. For example, a book on leadership skills may identify core abilities in the opening chapter, and then examine each one in detail. There is no right or wrong about how you order your material. The main requirement is that ideas are arranged logically so that related material is placed together in a coherent fashion.

You will have a target word length that you have agreed with the publisher. The allocation of words to each chapter or section is an important early stage in your planning. You may need to modify your estimates later on, as you do more research and start writing. However, it is a useful way of avoiding pitfalls such as using up half of your word allowance on the first two chapters.

It can be hard to take an overview of the contents when you are dealing with so much information. However, it is vital to do this so that you avoid repetition, inconsistencies and omissions. One method is to use large A3 paper to record the content. Write out the key points from each chapter or section in a similar order to how you plan to write them in the book. Use at least one sheet per chapter. Sticking them on the wall like posters makes it easier to see and compare each one.

All writers agree that the hardest task is sitting down and getting the words down on paper. They will also say that writing involves a process of review and revision. You are likely to have to make several drafts before you are happy with the final product. Reviewing your writing regularly helps improve your writing style, and keeps you on track if you also monitor how it compares with your original goals. It is often very helpful to leave your work for several weeks before rereading it. You will have a fresher eye and editing will be much easier. The action points at the end of this chapter offer a few tips on how to get started and to keep going with your writing.

**Presenting your manuscript**

You will need to prepare your manuscript for submission. See Chapter 18 'Presenting Your Work' for more detailed advice or refer to your publisher's guidelines.

The usual arrangement of a manuscript is:

- ○ Title page
- ○ (Special notes)
- ○ (Acknowledgements)
- ○ Contents page
- ○ Foreword
- ○ Main text (in order of the chapters or sections)
- ○ Figures (collated in the order in which they appear in the text)
- ○ Notes (collated in the same way as figures)
- ○ Reference list
- ○ Bibliography
- ○ Appendices.

The publishing process after the submission of your final manuscript usually follows these stages:

1. The manuscript is checked by the commissioning editor who may return it to you if any revisions are required. You will need to agree and make any necessary changes or additions.

2. Your manuscript will also be seen by a copy-editor who will check that it conforms to the publisher's house style. A list of any queries will be sent to you, and the manuscript will be amended according to your responses.

3.  Once the queries have been dealt with, your manuscript becomes the final agreed draft. This is sent to the production department for the design work and preparation for typesetting.

4.  Proofs are prepared once your manuscript has been typeset. These are sent to you for checking against the agreed final draft. Your responsibility as an author is to check for errors. Do not attempt to rewrite or insert additional material at this stage. Changes once a manuscript has been typeset are costly and may delay publication. Any alterations not in the agreed final draft will almost certainly have to be paid for by you. This is why it is essential to have completed and thoroughly checked your manuscript before you agree it as the final draft.

5.  Once the proofs have been dealt with, the next stage is printing the book. Your publisher should be able to give you some idea of the timescale for this. You can then sit back and await the immense satisfaction of seeing your work in print.

## Action Points

### (A) Ten tips to beat writer's block!

1.  Make a writing space for yourself. A whole room as a study is ideal but not always feasible. Instead find a corner that you can make your own and use only for writing. In this way you will start to make a psychological link between this place and the act of writing.

2.  Write a set amount of words each day or each session. The most important thing is to get something down on paper. The aim is to establish a writing habit – something you do every day. You will then find that you have a piece of work you can refine and develop, rather than a blank piece of paper.

3.  Watch out for 'perfectionism'. Avoid agonising over every word and every sentence.

4.  Think before you commit yourself to paper. You may falter in your writing due to a lack of information or an unclear plan.

5.  Break the task down into manageable pieces. Write in short blocks with a specific goal in mind, such as completing a section or writing a summary.

6.  Take a break from your writing. It often helps to put your writing to one side for a period of time. You will be fresher in your review when you come back to it at a later stage.

7.  Make sure you plan optimum writing times. Choose the time of day when you are most energetic. Work in blocks of 45 minutes. It will be at least 20 minutes before you are fully focused on the task. Any longer than an hour and your concentration will start to decline. Give yourself five-minute breaks in between blocks.

8.  Finish each writing session on a high note. Stop when your writing is going well, not when you are beginning to struggle with it. Try to leave a small but achievable task undone. You will then have something to do immediately at the start of your next session, for instance writing out a list or putting in headings.

9.  Set yourself a time limit and stick to it. Work often expands to fit the time available. Instead give yourself a deadline to complete specific tasks.

10. Reward yourself each time you reach one of your goals. Try small rewards for your small goals and a very big reward for meeting one of your major goals.

### (B) Start preparing information for the book cover

You will be asked by the publisher to give two main pieces of information. First a description of yourself ('the author') and second, a description of the book.

### Description of the author

Your publisher will require a brief résumé about yourself and any co-authors. This information will be used by the publisher in any advertising material and will also appear on the book cover. Details might include:

- your full name, title and details of qualifications
- your present job title and place of employment if you want this to be included
- three or four lines of information about you that will be of interest to the reader – this will include any experience or knowledge that qualifies you to write on the subject of your book.

*Description of the book*

Try to include:

- the intended readership (for example, undergraduates, postgraduate students, practitioners, specific disciplines)
- the reason for the book (for example, to help deal with changes in the structure of the NHS service, to update clinical knowledge or skills, to meet the growing demand for information by clients)
- the style of the book (for example, easy-to-use handbook, case study format)
- any special characteristics of the book (for example, combines text with video, is in A to Z format, features a CD-ROM).

---

### Summary Points

- Decide on the topic, scope, aims, approach and intended readership of your book before you approach a publisher.
- Check that your book is different enough from other complementary or competitive texts to have a place in the book market.
- Find a publisher who will be interested in your type of book, and make contact with them initially by letter. Include a synopsis of your book that outlines its aims, approach and content.

---

- ○ Most publishers at some stage require a written proposal. This will include information not only on your book but also on the target market.

- ○ Writing a book follows similar stages to other types of composition. You will need to plan, research, draft, edit, and prepare your final draft for submission.

- ○ Once your manuscript has been submitted there may be queries from the commissioning editor and the copy-editor. You will need to respond to these before you can agree a final draft to go forward to the production department.

- ○ The cost of any alterations or additions to the manuscript once it has been typeset and proofs prepared is usually borne by the author.

# 22

# Articles for the Media

Health and the health care system are favourite topics for the media. Any edition of a popular newspaper or magazine is likely to carry at least one article on the subject. This is partly due to the fact that people are increasingly interested in finding out how to have a healthy lifestyle. They want to be active in the prevention of ill health, and to know about the illnesses that may already affect them personally.

Attention is also focused on the roles and responsibilities of various health professionals. This is reflected in the growing number of 'day in the life' type of features. Readers are curious about the tasks facing staff in their everyday working life. They are keen to know about the personal characteristics and professional skills required to deal with often challenging situations.

**Why write for the media?**
Writing an article or feature for a newspaper or magazine is one way of fulfilling the creative urge to write. However, there are also a number of sound professional reasons for getting published in this way. Articles can help to:

- increase the profile of your discipline in the public eye
- raise awareness of a particular condition or disease
- assist in educating the public about a healthy lifestyle
- focus on the causes and manifestations of specific ailments and the treatment options that are available
- provide information on a new treatment or a new type of service

- provide advice for readers on how to cope with the consequences of specific illnesses and the side effects of treatment

- boost fundraising by featuring a special event

- offer a forum for you to express a personal opinion on a topical issue.

**Aspects of writing for the media**

Writing an article for the media differs significantly from writing an academic paper or journal article. Here are a few aspects you need to consider.

Your readership will have limited knowledge and experience of the topic. This will affect your choice of language and the type and amount of information you give.

Messages given via the media have a greater impact than other forms of communication. It is essential that information is accurate, up to date and not alarmist.

The need to sell copies is an overriding concern for the media. This will influence the content, style and perspective of the publication. Articles often take a certain slant or angle on a topic in order to attract the interest of specific readers. This will be reflected in the emphasis and approach of the articles. You need to consider this carefully when choosing a publication for your article.

Time is a crucial factor when preparing any article for publication. It is even more of a consideration when writing for magazines and newspapers. Planning, particularly for magazines, is usually done several months ahead. Newspapers might have a relatively short preparation time. This needs to be taken into consideration if your work needs to be published by a certain date.

Remember:

- Client confidentiality must be maintained at all times. This is not just about readers identifying the client, but also about the client being able to identify himself or herself. This can be equally damaging and distressing.

- You will need to seek permission from your manager and employing organisation if your article relates in any way to your employment.

### What are you going to write about?

Before you get started you will need to have some basic ideas about:

- the subject or topic you want to write about (see Chapter 14 'Developing an Idea' to help give you some inspiration)

- who you are writing it for (your intended readership)

- your market or where you might publish (local or national newspaper, weekly or monthly magazine, generalist or specialist journal)

- whether you will supply illustrations (see Chapter 18 'Presenting Your Work' on the use of illustrations).

You are more likely to be successful if you write your article for a specific magazine or newspaper – so before you finalise your idea, try to identify the most appropriate publication for your needs.

### Finding a market

Each newspaper or magazine is designed, written and presented in a way that will attract certain groups of the population. Many will have a national distribution and contain articles and features of interest to a broad section of readers. Others are restricted to a regional or local circulation area. There are also many specialist publications that maintain a small but well-defined readership.

All these things need to be taken into consideration when deciding which newspaper or magazine you would like to approach. For example, a local or regional newspaper may be a better choice if you are hoping to do some fundraising for health provision within your local community. An article on health promotion would receive a greater audience in a national paper.

You can find out more about the aims, content and readership of various newspapers and magazines by consulting one of the directories or guides on this subject. The following books provide a wealth of information about the market in these media:

- *The Writer's Handbook*

- *Willings Press Guide*

- *Writers' & Artists' Yearbook.*

They will also give you information about which publications will consider freelance contributions. Some major newspapers and magazines either use in-house staff or only commission pieces from established journalists. Seek out those publications that have indicated that they consider external contributors.

Supplement information from the above guides by doing your own research. Make sure that you have read at least three recent issues of the publication.

- What topics are usually featured?

- Does the article have a particular angle or slant?

- Is this a characteristic of the whole publication? For instance, one magazine may be interested in alternative or unusual health remedies, whereas another may favour a more traditional account of treatment and therapy.

- How much detail is included? Monthly or quarterly magazines usually have longer and more in-depth articles than weeklies.

Compare how the same topic is treated in different publications:

- What aspects of the topic have been highlighted? (One magazine may provide a detailed report containing facts and figures on the growth of alcoholism in young people. Another may choose to take a more upbeat approach, and focus on how families can recognise and help adolescents who have a drink problem.)

- How has the topic been approached? For example, it might be from a personal perspective. The reader is taken on a journey through the development of an illness as seen and felt by an individual with this condition. It may be focused on the illness itself with descriptions and explanations presented in a clinical and detached manner.

- What style has been used – practical and straightforward, detailed and academic, conversational or narrative?

Editors will be looking for items that will be of interest to their readers. Therefore it is essential that your piece also fulfils this criterion if it is to be accepted. Your market research must include a study of the needs and concerns of your intended audience. You will have gained some insight about the readers by looking at the type of features in the paper or magazine.

Remember that you can also build up a profile of the reader by looking at the advertisements (Dick 1996). What are the adverts trying to sell? Who would be most likely to buy the products they advertise? What type of person is portrayed in the adverts? Other clues will come from the letters page or similar slots where the reader is able to contribute. What are the main interests expressed through these pages? Are there any queries or comments regarding health matters? The answers to these questions will tell you, amongst other things, the age range, educational level, and social and economic grouping of the readership.

Find out how long the publication needs for preparing articles for publication. This is known as the lead time and will vary between magazines and newspapers. You need to be sure that you have time to write the article and prepare it for submission.

At the end of your research, you will know:

- the circulation of the publication
- how often it is published
- the lead time
- the target readership
- the aims of the publication
- the type of articles
- the general approach of the publication
- the style of presentation.

You will now be able to make a shortlist of magazines or papers you wish to approach. Remember that a successful submission will conform to the usual style, tone and content of the publication.

### Making an approach

It is important to only contact one paper or magazine at a time, so start with the publication that is top of your list. Make your approach in writing. This gives you time to prepare what you want to say and put forward your ideas in the best way. Although some editors are prepared to read through unsolicited manuscripts, the majority prefer authors to send a preliminary letter containing a synopsis of their proposed article. This is usually referred to as a query letter, and will save you committing time to writing the whole article until you have at least a firm indication of interest. Address your letter to the appropriate editor. This information is sometimes given in the writing guides (listed earlier) or you may be able to find it in an issue of the publication.

A query letter needs to be concise and include such details as:

- A few brief introductory details about yourself. (Include any information that shows you have the relevant expertise to write the article, for example your occupation, professional qualifications, any previous writing experience. Remember you are selling yourself as well as your article.)

- A synopsis – this is a summary of your article. It will give the editor an idea of the content and the style of presentation.

- A statement about how you think your contribution will suit the approach of the magazine and meet the needs of its readers.

- A description of any illustrations you may be able to provide. (Do not send any at this stage.)

See Figure 22.1 for an example of a query letter.

Remember to include a stamped addressed envelope for a reply. It may be several weeks before you hear anything so be patient and definitely avoid the temptation to canvass other editors.

You are likely to get one of the following responses:

- A definite acceptance. Great! You can go ahead and agree terms. (See the Chapter 19 'Protecting Your Rights' for advice on contracts.)

- An expression of interest, but the editor has some queries in terms of content or approach. This is a more likely response than an outright acceptance. You now have the option to negotiate and rework your piece until you have a mutually acceptable idea. (Once you have agreed an idea it should not be radically changed without discussion with the editor.)

- A clear and firm rejection. This can be very disheartening. However, a negative response is not necessarily a sign that your proposal is at fault.

Rochelle Merrow-Hart
12a Barking Street
Rochester
Kent
ME1 7TU

21/3/2001

Diane Justin
Editor
Healthy Baby Magazine
131-133 Pickering Avenue
London
W1 ENR

Dear Diane Justin,

I am a practising midwife and lecturer in midwifery. I have enclosed an outline of an article on planning a home delivery. It will be approximately 1500 words in length.

I feel this practical article will fit with your magazine's modern approach to childbirth. It provides advice on planning a home delivery and includes two case studies.

I have previously had articles published in the Midwifes Association Newsletter and Parentcraft Journal.

I enclose a stamped addressed envelope for your reply.

I look forward to hearing from you.

Yours sincerely,


Signature
Name (title/qualifications)
Position

*Figure 22.1 A query letter*

Check out the reason why your idea has not been accepted. Always consider any advice or comments from the editor. Is the idea basically sound but is it not what the editor is looking for at the present time? Has the topic already been covered, or is it not one the editor feels will interest his or her readership? Is the style unsuitable for the publication? Answers to these questions will help you decide whether you need to modify your style, approach or content.

If you still think your idea is good, then move quickly on to another publication and start the process all over again. Whatever happens, remember – a rejection at this stage, before you have written an entire article, will save you time and effort.

## Writing your article

It is worth spending time studying how media articles are written and constructed. You will find that like any other piece of writing, each one will have a typical three-part structure. This consists of the introduction, the main body and the conclusion.

### *The introduction*

Introductions tend to be brief with the topic and the author's perspective on it quickly conveyed to the reader. Read the introduction to different articles that deal with similar subject matter: how did you know what the content would be? What angle did the writer take? How was this conveyed – by the tone, style or choice of words? Check that your introduction clearly indicates your topic and signals the perspective you will be taking.

### *The main body*

The main body of the article will contain the bulk of the information.

### *Content*

Compare the content of different articles on the same topic:

- List the key messages.
- Look at the facts, examples and analogies supporting each of these main points. How much detail was included?
- How were the points linked together?
- What information was included?
- What information was omitted?

- What was achieved by the end of the article (an increase in understanding, a greater insight, knowledge of a practical skill)?

Your planning will help you decide on your main messages. Think about what the reader will want to know. What are the most frequently asked questions on this topic? What aspects of the topic will be of interest to the target readers? Is there anything new or controversial you wish to cover?

Make a note of examples, explanations and so on that you will use to support your main points. Write these down alongside the key points in your plan.

Once you have a basic outline of your article, you can start thinking about how you will present the content.

When giving information:

- Make sure it is accurate.

- Make sure it is up to date with new developments.

- Avoid being alarmist.

When giving instructions about practical matters:

- Break the information down into more manageable chunks – for example, what equipment you need, when to do it and step by step instructions.

- Make the sequence of actions clear – use bullet points or step one, two and so on.

- Use illustrations to help the reader visualise the process.

- Get a lay person to read your draft and comment – or, better still, ask him or her to follow your instructions and see what happens. Remember even a very simple sequence of actions is hard to convey in a concise manner. Try writing down instructions for tying your shoelaces!

When explaining terminology or procedures:

- Use simple and straightforward language.

- Be careful not to confuse the reader by using unfamiliar medical terms in your explanation.

Information boxes are frequently used in media articles. These are boxed or shaded areas containing text written in the form of bullet points. They help direct the reader's attention to key information. Consider how you might use these information boxes in your article.

When giving advice try:

- Top Tips
- Helpful Hints
- Five Ways to Help
- Three Golden Rules
- Dos and Don'ts
- If you...

When giving information try:

- It's a Fact
- Did you know...?
- Lists (for example, symptoms, causes).

When challenging assumptions and false beliefs:

- True or False?
- Fact or Fiction?
- Beliefs and Myths.

When providing guidelines on seeking professional help:

- Five Reasons to Call a Doctor
- Warning Signs
- If you are worried...
- You need help if...
- Seek help when...

Be careful not to overuse boxes. The majority of information still needs to be in the main text.

### Length

Space is at a premium in newspapers and magazines. Articles must be fitted around the important income-generating advertisements. This means it is essential to stay within the agreed word length.

Part of your planning will involve working out how many words you want to allocate to each section of your work. As you start to write you may find that you have to adapt your plan so that some sections are longer and others shorter.

If you find that you have strayed over the word length, try to edit your work so that it is more concise. For example, 'your headings' uses fewer words than 'the headings you use in your manuscript' but still retains the meaning. However, if this is not possible you will have to consider omitting some of the content itself. Select minor details that do not affect the overall meaning of the piece.

### Structure

Study how articles are arranged. Most will use headings to provide a framework for the text. Look at how these are used to help the reader.

In general, headings help:

- to provide a framework
- to break the text into shorter and more manageable sections for the reader
- as signposts to help the reader find specific information
- to signal a change in topic
- to help the flow of the article.

Choose your headings and write your content around these. However, be aware that the editor may need to change your headings in order to fit your piece into the available space.

### Style

Media articles usually have an easy-to-read style. This is often achieved by the use of short sentences written in the active rather than the passive voice. Aim to keep your sentences simple, with a maximum of 20 words.

Remember you are writing for a lay audience. This will influence your choice of language and the way in which you express ideas. You will not be able to assume an underlying knowledge base in the same way that you can when writing for other professionals. However, the reader will have some understanding of health matters. For example, you may safely assume that many female readers will understand the term 'oestrogen', but they may need an explanation of 'androgens'.

The age, gender and culture of the reader are also important factors. For example, an article about contraceptives in a teenage magazine will require more explanation than one aimed at women in their thirties.

### The conclusion
The conclusion helps to bring the article to a close. Look at various articles and compare the opening paragraph with the last. You will find that the concluding comments often relate in some way to the introduction. This helps to give the reader a sense of completeness.

The end of the article is also the place for details such as other sources of information, advice or support. Include any contact addresses and telephone numbers for associations, helplines or self-help groups.

### Presentation and submission of your article
Always follow the publication's guidelines for preparing and submitting your manuscript. (See Chapter 18 'Presenting Your Work' for more information.)

### Action Points

1. Use a checklist to help you research newspapers and magazines. Read at least three recent copies of your target newspaper or magazine. Use the guide in Figure 22.2 to help you analyse the content, approach and style.

| | |
|---|---|
| What is the circulation? | ° Check the relevant guides |
| How often is it published? | ° Check the relevant guide<br>° Check magazine or newspaper |
| Who are the target readers? | ° Read relevant guides<br>° Read features/articles<br>° Look at advertisements<br>° Check contributors to the letters page |
| What are the aims of the publication? | ° Read relevant guides<br>° Read editor's comments<br>° Check guidelines for submission |

| | |
|---|---|
| What types of articles appear in the publication? | ❏ News stories<br>❏ Regular series<br>❏ General interest features<br>❏ Specialist features<br>❏ Science articles<br>❏ Technical articles<br>❏ Lifestyle articles<br>❏ Travel features<br>❏ Personal accounts<br>❏ Nostalgia items<br>❏ Humorous clips<br>❏ Profiles<br>❏ Events<br>❏ Letters |
| What is the general approach of the publication? | ❏ Aimed at male/female/<br>   adolescents/children<br>❏ Traditional<br>❏ Family orientated<br>❏ General interest<br>❏ Glamorous<br>❏ Intellectual<br>❏ Topical<br>❏ Trendy<br>❏ Controversial |
| What is the style of presentation? | ° Average word length _____<br>° Type of vocabulary<br>_____<br>° Complexity of material<br>_____ |

*Figure 22.2 A guide to analysing the content, approach and style of media articles*

2. Think about newspaper and magazine articles you have read. Which ones did you like? Why? Make a note of their good and bad points. How could they have been improved?

## Summary Points

- Writing articles for the media can help to raise the profile of your profession as well as providing information for the general public.

- Remember to seek permission from your employers if you are writing about your employment or organisation.

- Obtain consent to use information about clients and ensure confidentiality is maintained.

- Articles written for a specific magazine or newspaper are more likely to be successful. Identify an appropriate publication before you start to write.

- Remember that media publications have an overriding concern to sell copies and may have a specific angle or slant. You need to consider this carefully when choosing a publication.

- Make your approach to the editor using a preliminary letter containing a synopsis of your proposed article.

- Find out how far in advance of publication you need to submit your article.

- Your readers are a lay audience with a limited knowledge and experience of the topic. This will affect your choice of language and the type and amount of information you give.

- Make sure information is accurate and up to date. Avoid being alarmist.

- Use information boxes to give key points.

- Keep to the agreed word length as space is at a premium in newspapers and magazines.

# References

*Abortion Act* (1967). London: HMSO.

*Abortions Regulations* (1991). London: HMSO.

*Access to Health Records Act* (1990). London: HMSO.

Albert, T. and Chadwick, S. (1992) 'How Readable are Practice Leaflets.' *British Medical Journal* 305, 1266–1268.

ALBSU (1992) *Making Reading Easier.* London: The Adult Literacy and Basic Skills Unit.

Audit Commission (1993) *What Seems to be the Matter: Communication Between Hospitals and Patients.* London: HMSO.

Audit Commission (1995) *Setting the Records Straight: A Study of Medical Records.* London: HMSO.

Austoker, J. and Ong, G. (1994) 'Written Information Needs of Women who are Recalled for Further Investigation of Breast Screening: Results of a Multicentre Study.' *Journal of Medical Screening* 1, 238–244.

Barnes, R. (1995) *Successful Study for Degrees* (2nd edition). London: Routledge.

Bligh, D. (1983) *What's the use of Lectures?* Harmondsworth, Middlesex: Penguin.

Brown, G. (1978) *'Lecturing and Explaining'.* London: Methuen.

Burnett, J. (1979) *Successful Study: A Handbook for Students.* Sevenoaks, Kent: Hodder & Stoughton.

Buzan, T. (1989) *Use Your Head.* London: BBC Books.

*Caldicott Report* (1997). London: NHS Executive.

*Children's Act* (1989). London: HMSO.

Churchill Livingstone (1996) *Guide for Authors.* Edinburgh: Pearson Professional Ltd.

Cohen, W.I. (1983) 'Establishing Effective Parent/Patient Communication.' In M. King, L. Novak and C. Citrenbaum *Irresistible Communication: Creative Skills for the Health Professional.* London: W.B. Saunders.

Coulter, A., Entwistle, V. and Gilbert, D. (1998) *Informing Patients: An Assessment of the Quality of Patient Information Materials.* London: King's Fund Publishing.

*Data Protection Act* (1998). London: HMSO.

Department of Health (1995) *'The Patient's Charter' and You* (1995) London: HMSO.

Department of Health (2001) *NHS Plan.* London: HMSO.

Dick, J. (1996) *Writing for Magazines* (2nd edition). London: A & C Black Publishing Ltd.

Dimond, B. (2000) 'Legal Issues Arising in Community Nursing 3: Consent and Compulsion.' *British Journal of Community Nursing 5,* 1, 32–33.

Doak, C., Doak, L. and Root, J. (1996) *Teaching Patients with Low Literacy Skills* (2nd edition). Philadelphia: J.B. Lippincott Co.

Dobson, A. (1995) *How to Write Business Letters (A Practical Introduction for Everyone).* Plymouth: How To Books Ltd.

Dorner, J. (1992) *Writing on Disk.* Hertfordshire: John Taylor Book Ventures.

Duman, M. and Farrell, C. (2000) *The Poppi Guide (Practicalities of Producing Patient Information).* London: King's Fund Publishing.

Ellis, D.A., Hopkins, J.M., Leitch, A.G. and Crofton, J. (1979) 'Doctor's Orders: Controlled Trial of Supplementary Written Information for Patients.' *British Medical Journal* 1, 456.

*Family Law Reform Act* (1969). London: HMSO.

Fisher, M. (2001) 'Educational Input to Improve Documentation Skills.' *Nursing Times* 97, 8, 35–36.

Flesch, R. (1948) 'A New Readability Yardstick.' *Journal of Applied Psychology 32,* 3, 221–223.

Flesch, R. (1964) *How to Write, Speak & Think More Effectively.* New York: Signet Books.

French, P. (1994) *Social Skills for Nursing Practice* (2nd edition). London: Chapman & Hall.

Garratt, S. (1985) *Managing Your Time.* London: Fontana.

Gibbs, G. (1981) 'Twenty Terrible Reasons for Lecturing.' Paper No. 8. Birmingham: Standing Conference in Educational Development.

Gibbs, G. (1992) 'Teaching More Students: Number 2 Lecturing to More Students.' Oxford. The Polytechnics and Colleges Funding Council.

Gunning, R. (1952) *The Teaching of Clear Writing.* New York: McGraw-Hill.

Hartley, J. (1980) *The Psychology of Written Communication.* London: Kogan Press.

*Health Act* (1999). London: HMSO.

*Human Fertilisation and Embryology (Disclosure of Information) Act* (1992). London: HMSO.

Inglis, J. and Lewis, R. (1982) *Report Writing (The Secret of Successful Reports).* Cambridge: National Extension College.

King, M., Novak, L. and Citrenbaum, C. (1983) *Irresistible Communication: Creative Skills for the Health Professional.* London: W. B. Saunders.

Krenter, M.W., Bull, F.C., Clark, E.M. and Oswald, L. (1999) 'Understanding How People Process Health Information: A Comparison of Tailored and Non-tailored Weight Loss Materials.' *Health Psychology 18*, 5, 487–494.

Leader, W.G. (1990) *How to Pass Exams.* Cheltenham: Stanley Thomas Publishers Ltd.

Ley, P. (1982) 'Studies of Recall in Medical Settings.' *Human Learning 1* 223–33.

Ley, P. (1988) *Communicating with Patients (Improving Communication, Satisfaction and Compliance).* London: Chapman & Hall.

*Mental Health Act* (1983). London: HMSO.

Moody, M. (2001) 'Why Nurses End Up in Court'. *Nursing Times 97*, 8., 24–26.

National Health Service Executive (1990) *Consent to Treatment and Examination* (Appendix B). London: NHS Executive.

National Health Service Executive (1996) *The Protection and Use of Patient Information.* Health Service Guidelines (96)18/LASSL(96)5. London: NHS Executive.

National Health Service Executive (1998) *Preservation, Retention and Destruction of GP Medical Services Records Relating to Patients.* Health Service Circular 1998/217. London: NHS Executive.

National Health Service Executive (1999) *For the Record: Managing Records in NHS Trusts and Health Authorities.* Health Service Circular 1999/053. London: NHS Executive.

National Health Service Training Division (1994) *Just for the Record: A Guide to Record Keeping for Health Care Professionals.* London: Department of Health.

*NHS Trusts and Primary Care Trusts (Sexually Transmitted Diseases) Directions* (2000). London: Department of Health.

Newman, R. (1989) *Study and Research – A Systematic Approach for All Students.* Oxford: Bookmarque Publishing.

Ong, G., Austoker, J. and Brouwer, A. (1996) 'Evaluation of the Written Information Sent to Women who are Called Back for Further Investigation of Breast Screening in the UK.' *Health Education Journal 55*, 4, 413–429.

Pagano, M.P. and Ragan, S.L. (1992) *Communication Skills for Professional Nurses.* London: Sage Publications.

Pernet, R. (1989) *Effective Use of Time* (2nd edition). London: The Industrial Society.

Polit, D. and Hungler, B. (1995) *Essentials of Nursing Research: Methods, appraisal and utilization* (5th edition). Philadelphia, PA: Lippincott.

*Prevention of Terrorism Act* (1989). London: HMSO.

*Public Records Act* (1958). London: HMSO.

Quantum Development (2000) *Expert Evidence Toolbox.* Chorley, Lancs: Quantum Development.

Rodgers, M.E. (2000) 'The Child Patient and Consent to Treatment: Legal Overview.' *British Journal of Community Nursing 5,* 10, 494–498.

Shaw, L. (2001) 'Rights for All (The Human Rights Act – What Does it Mean for Us).' *CSLT Bulletin* (February) 14–15.

Shimoda, T.A. (1994) *Excellent Communication Skills Required for Engineering Managers.* New York: American Society of Civil Engineers.

Springhouse Corporation (1998) *Charting Made Incredibly Easy.* Pennsylvania: Springhouse.

Taylor, J. (1992) *Study Skills for Nurses.* London: Chapman & Hall.

*The Writer's Handbook.* (Revised annually.) London: Pan McMillan.

Togo, D. and Hood, J. (1992) 'Quantitative Information Presentation and Gender: An Interaction Effect' *The Journal of General Psychology 119,* 161–167.

White, J. (1987) 'The Journal Publication Process: The Perspective of the Nurse Author.' *Journal of Advanced Nursing 12,* 121–127.

*Willings Press Guide.* (Revised annually.) Bucks: Willings Press.

Winkler, A.C. and McCuen, J.R. (1999) *Writing the Research Paper – A Handbook.* London: Harcourt Brace College publishers.

Woodward, L. and Charlton, A. (1995) 'The British Medical Association TP Gunton Award 1995: Development of a Health Education Leaflet to Promote Early Detection of Oral Cancer.' *International Journal of Health Promotion & Education 37,* 1, 5–10.

World Cancer Research Fund (2000) '*Reducing Your Risk of Prostate Cancer.*' World Cancer Research Fund: London.

*Writers' & Artists' Yearbook.* (Revised annually.) London: A & C Black.

Young, L. and Humphrey, M. (1985) 'Cognitive Methods of Preparing Women for Hysterectomy: Does a Booklet Help?' *British Journal of Clinical Psychology 24,* 303–304.

# Index

Abstracts 281–282
Access to health records 32, 35,
38–40, 67
    restrictions on disclosure of
    information 39
Access to Health Records Act 1990
39
Accountability 34–35
Articles for the Media,
    aspects of writing for 303
    finding a market 304–306
    making an approach 306–308
    writing your article 309–313

Books,
    approaching a publisher
    290–291
    checking the market 290
    presenting a manuscript 297–298
    proposal 291–295
    writing 295–297

Caldicott Report 35
Care pathways (clinical pathways)
54–55, 96, 126
Care plans
    definition 54,
    evaluation 63–64
    implementation 62–63
    setting measurable goals 59–61
    writing interventions 61–62
    writing objectives 54–56, 58–61
Co-authors 256–289
Conclusions 73, 84, 137–138, 174,
178–179, 205, 208
Confidentiality
    obtaining 35–39
    children and young people
    36–37
    exceptions 37
    protecting 208, 284, 303
Consent,
    to disclosure of information 36
    obtaining 47, 56–58

recording 52, 57, 64, 69
    young people 36–37, 38,
Contemporaneous records 32
Contracts 272–273
Copyright 270–271

Database 125, 127–130, 162, 234,
254, 281
Data Protection Act 1994 39
Data Protection Act 1998 29–30, 34,
35, 36, 39–40, 87
Disks 255–256, 266
Displaying numerical information
210–218
Dissertations,
    structure 196–197
    title 194,196
    topic 195–196

Effective Reading 130–134
Essays,
    assessment criteria 179–183
    planning 168–174
    submission 183–184
    writing 174–184
Explanations 134–136, 149, 249

Finding information 124–126
Function of written language 11

Illustrations 106, 264–265, 304,
307, 310
Internet 125, 126, 127, 128, 254
Introductions 72–73, 82–83,134,
174–176, 282–283, 309

Journal Articles,
    approaching a journal 278
    submitting an article 284–285
    writing an article 278–282

Letters,
    lay-out 74–75
    purpose 23–24
    structure 72–74
    types of,71, 80–82

writing 77–80
Libraries 126–127, 128

Mind maps 188–189

Note taking,
  lectures 161–162
  organising notes 163–164
  purpose 153–154
  pattern notes 159–160
  practical demonstrations 163
  sequential notes 155–157
  spider notes 157–159
  text 162–163

Patient's Charter 36
Personal health records,
  definition 21
  purpose 21–23
  retention 40–42, 67
  security 37–38
  setting up 45–46

Quotes 136, 263

Recording,
  casehistory 48 –49
  consent 57
  contacts 44–45
  discharge 51–52, 65–67, 70,
    90–91
  initial assessment 47–53
  intervention 53–65
  referrals 46–47, 49, 53, 69, 81,
    90
References 197–203
Reports,
  format 82–84
  purpose 24 –25, 86
  types 90–91
  writing 85–90
Research papers,
  quantative 205
  qualitative 208
Revision 123, 153–154, 160, 166,
  188–189

Royalties 273

Searches 96, 127–130, 195
Summaries 52, 96, 137

Teaching Materials,
  delivering the message 142–143
  evaluation 151
  flipcharts 148–149
  handouts 149–150
  overhead projector 144–146
  planning 141
  slide projector 146–147
  whiteboard 147–148

Use of colour 107–110, 144, 157,
  159–160, 164

Writer's Block 298–299
Written materials for clients,
  delivering the message 97
  evaluation 114–116
  improving recall of information
    102–104
  increasing comprehension
    100–101
  illustrations 106
  planning content 94–96
  purpose 25–27
  story boards 96
  team approach 93–94
  typography 104–106
written materials for special clients,
  English as a second language
    112–114
  literacy difficulties 109–112
  sensory impairment 114